Living Forever Chic

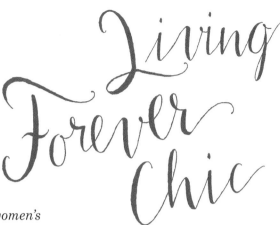

Living Forever Chic

Frenchwomen's
  Timeless Secrets for
Everyday Elegance,
  Gracious Entertaining,
and Enduring Allure

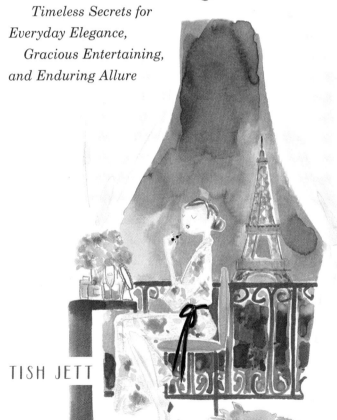

TISH JETT

Rizzoli
ex libris

DEDICATION

For my darling Ella

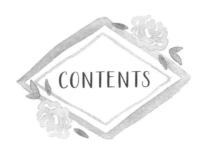

CONTENTS

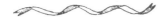

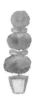

INTRODUCTION

How—and Why—to Live Forever Chic

With each passing birthday, I realize that one of the most important goals in my life is serenity. I want serene surroundings and relationships. I want my wardrobe pared down and useful for all occasions, my makeup and skin care efficacious, and my home a lovely, soothing, well-organized sanctuary. In other words, I want my life to run as smoothly, beautifully, and effortlessly as it would for a Frenchwoman of a certain age.

The French have a phrase for this. (Of course they do. The French have a phrase for everything.) *L'art de vivre*, which means, in essence, a life well lived. *L'art de vivre* à *la française* covers everything from the way one should conduct oneself to how to dress, entertain, decorate, and maintain a home. When we decide to consciously cultivate and celebrate *l'art de vivre,* our lives become richer and more fulfilling. The components of *l'art de vivre* permeate every aspect of life, from ingrained respect for others and *les bonnes manières* to entertaining, dressing, and decorating.

My first book, *Forever Chic*, focused on what we could learn from Frenchwomen of a certain age regarding beauty, fashion, diet, and exercise. In this book, I've broadened the notion of living well, making it my goal to discover how Frenchwomen of a certain age apply the principles of *l'art de vivre* in their lives. They are, after all, the ones who set the example for the next generation (as well as their partners), as their mothers, aunts, and grandmothers did before them. They are the historians of family traditions and their cultural heritage. With their quiet examples of grace and refinement, they have always been a great inspiration to me.

While many aspects of life are beyond our control, there are always life-enhancing details that are totally *within* our control. No one understands this better than *les femmes françaises d'un certain age*. Over the years, my friends and I have evolved from young women with young children into mothers of adults of the same ages we were when we first met. Now we're undeniably women of a certain age, and many of us are grandmothers, all of which adds another dimension of happiness and purpose to our lives.

Over my many years of living in France and observing these women, I've learned how even the smallest attention to detail makes an enormous difference in the pleasure and beauty we can bring into our daily lives. I've found in emulating the remarkable discipline my French friends and acquaintances apply to their lives, those small daily habits of taking good care of themselves and their homes, contentment and a peaceful sense of joy result.

As I've said many times, discipline will set us free. Consciously deciding to ward off chaos by doing such simple tasks as maintaining a well-arranged closet;

crafting an intelligent and functional wardrobe; polishing silver, unless you're a fan of the unpolished look, which some Frenchwomen like; organizing a logical (and sweetly perfumed) linen closet; having cooking staples ever present in the kitchen and the freezer, so there is always something on hand to throw together a quick meal; creating a clutter-free living room with pretty, comfortable furniture—all so simple, and yet without these small but continuous efforts, our lives would slide into disarray.

Yes, our schedules are often complicated with obligations and demands that absorb our days and sap our energy. Time is a precious luxury, and saving it can become a priority. Who among us hasn't felt that it takes too much time and effort to make a real meal? That's why pizza was invented, but that doesn't mean the box goes on the dining table. Simply add cloth napkins, pretty place mats, and something decorative to the center of the dinner table, along with a no-fuss salad and the dressing that you made in advance over the weekend, and a civilized meal is on the table in less than ten minutes.

What Frenchwomen know from experience is that we can design our own lifestyles and create pleasing and pleasurable environments and experiences.

Organization is key. Discipline is necessary.

In my last book, *Forever Chic*, I wrote about my best French friend, Anne-Françoise de Saint Saëns-Henner, mother of six and now grandmother of thirteen, mistress of two exquisite homes, and sometime interior decorator, who has been from the moment we met (just months after my daughter and I arrived in France) my muse. When I would rave about the perfect order in her homes, she would simply say, "If I didn't keep everything in order, I could never enjoy my life. I have to be disciplined, otherwise I would have no time for myself. I would have no time to sit here and drink a glass of wine and chat with you."

What about the way we present ourselves to the world? We can be stylish and confident if we learn and accept the fact that Frenchwomen of a certain age know so well—that dressing well, in ways that manifest our personalities and our intentions, is *never* in direct correlation to our age, the amount of clothes we own, or how much they cost, but rather about how carefully and thoughtfully we choose items that are perfectly flattering for us. There is a world of difference in how I feel when I've pulled myself together with one of my favorite sweater-scarf-trouser and ballet flats combinations, nails polished, makeup, hair behaving itself, and perfume as opposed to sitting about in sweats with my hair in a messy ponytail, regardless of whether I leave the house. Furthermore, at this stage of our lives, we probably have our go-to "uniforms" in place so that dressing is easy. I know I do, and they are major confidence boosters. (For more on that subject, just in case we need to do a little work in our closets, please see Chapter 6: Le Style à la Française.) Dressing in a way that reflects our personal style is not complicated, and it's good for morale. You'll see; it's addictive.

> *"I don't want to look sloppy because then I feel sloppy."*
> —KARL LAGERFELD

Sometimes we might opt for the simple, at other times the enhanced, in all the areas of our lives from the way we dress and indulge in our beauty rituals to how we entertain and decorate our homes. No contradictions there. And what about our homes? We must not think that creating a calm, comfortable, charming oasis in our homes is a question of wherewithal any more than it is with our wardrobes. No matter what one's budget, living well is merely a question of desire and ingenuity. Gracious living is one of those little luxuries that delivers major rewards.

When I first started my career, I worked for a woman who told me to arrange my desk properly every evening before I left for the day, so that when I arrived the next morning, it would be welcoming. To this day, in my home office, I straighten up, even if it's simply arranging neat piles of notes and books. When I "come to work," I have the impression that I'm well organized.

In the chapters that follow, you'll see how scores of experts have added considerably more to the conversation about how we can cultivate not only *l'art de vivre*, but also elegance, *savoir faire*, and, as a result, *joie de vivre*. I've passed hours and hours with fashion icons, beauty experts, perfumers, Michelin two- and three-star chefs (as well as internationally acclaimed wine, cheese, and pastry masters), world-renowned hostesses, a talented florist, the art director of an haute couture linen house, interior designers, a landscape gardener, an authority on wearing and caring for cashmere, an absolutely hilarious observer and commentator on *le beau monde*, a professional protector and professor of *les bonnes manières*, and many others.

Within these pages, I'll show you what I've learned and how my life—and by extension, my daughter's life (she has transported what she learned as a child in France into her life in the United States)—has been enhanced by living in France. Since I am an American who has lived in France for more than thirty years, I am in that very special position of being an objective outside observer (or at least I try to be) in a culture that has radically changed my life in unexpected and positive ways. We are all capable of creating happiness and fulfillment every day in small and sometimes large ways, if we decide to make *l'art de vivre* and *joie de vivre* our priorities.

Please don't misunderstand me; I write about what I admire and appreciate in my French life from my point of view as a *femme d'un certain age*, but it is never my objective to set up an us-versus-them scenario. My intent is to share what I've learned and explain how I believe my life has been richer for the experience.

For those of us who may appreciate and aspire to certain aspects of *l'art de vivre à la française* but think it too rigorous, too time-consuming, or too complicated, let me show you that it is not. It's another one of those time equations with major dividends: Slight effort in equals major satisfaction and pleasure out.

Trust me, if I can get on board, anyone can.

So, once again, welcome to my world and thank you for joining me.

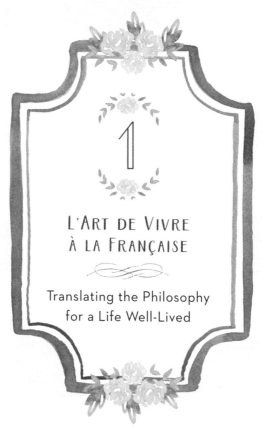

1

L'ART DE VIVRE
À LA FRANÇAISE

Translating the Philosophy
for a Life Well-Lived

Over the decades, Frenchwomen of a certain age have masterfully incorporated the fine art of living well into every aspect of their lives. They learned the importance of gracious living from their mothers and grandmothers and, I'm told, some from their great-grandmothers.

Family traditions and intergenerational respect live on today. I see it with my French niece, Alexandra, now in her fifties with three adult daughters and two grandchildren. Sunday lunches, holidays, vacations ... all revolve equally around the comfort and pleasure of the senior members of her family—now only her mother-in-law—and the fun element for younger members of the tribe. As extended family, we relish the excitement of being included in these festive moments.

As you have no doubt ascertained, I am fascinated by the universally understood aesthetic the French call *l'art de vivre*. Every Frenchwoman of a certain age that I know, and everyone I interviewed, agreed that it is the formula for experiencing a rich, fulfilling existence—not at all constraining, but rather liberating.

The translation of *l'art de vivre* is slightly more complex than the literal "art of living" phrase it translates to—which, when you think about it, doesn't offer sufficient useful information.

No, in French, *l'art de vivre* means celebrating and benefiting from the abundance of riches that each season and each day has to offer if we are consciously attuned to the world around us.

It is a reflection of tradition steeped in *une certaine manière d'être* (a certain way of being). French culture encompasses family, gastronomy, decoration, *l'art de table*, love of nature, gallantry, elegance, and an innate appreciation of quality in all things, from everyday goods like cheese and butter to luxury items like perfume and jewels.

Then there is the individual, very personal display of *l'art de vivre à la française* that has become synonymous the world over as displayed by Frenchwomen, particularly those of a certain age, who in so many ways represent the quintessential examples of charm, *les bonnes manières*, courtesy, refinement, and poise. Frenchwomen of a certain age perpetuate *l'art de vivre* by learning and applying a certain *savoir faire*, perfectly translated as "the ability to act and speak appropriately on all occasions." By definition, that includes respect, discretion, and kindness. For example, the Frenchwomen I know are the ultimate diplomats. Realizing that every family includes one or more "difficult" relations, they treat them with a delicate politesse and gently rebuff any unpleasant remark as if they didn't understand the intent. It's quite amazing to see.

The absolutely stunning fortysomething Camille Miceli, creative director of jewelry for Louis Vuitton, has a refreshing take on *l'art de vivre*. "It's an intellectual liberty," she says. "It's having the courage of your convictions, assuming your opinions and defending them, but always within the context of good manners and respect for others."

Over and over in my interviews, the importance of history was referenced in descriptions of *l'art de vivre,* and it became imminently clear that culture, custom, and references from the past are integral parts of the present and future that the French strive to protect. That is not to say that mores haven't evolved, that the French are not modern, innovative, and curious. *Au contraire.*

What other country had the vision and courage to elect a thirty-nine-year-old to lead them into the future? It was this mission that voters entrusted to Emmanuel Macron, the youngest president in the history of the country, on May 7, 2017. It is merely that they have the greatest respect for values that have endured.

President Macron's wife, Brigitte, is a stunning woman of a certain age (she is twenty-four years older than her husband) who reflects in her clothes and warm, open personality the very best of French elegance. The international press is enchanted by the couple's romantic complicity. I love watching them together.

WHAT *IS* IT ABOUT THE FRENCH?

The French have a complicated collective character that I can only explain as a mélange of hope and pragmatism. They are a philosophical lot. Like Socrates, they constantly pose questions. They question almost everything, often discuss minutiae beyond reason (in my opinion), philosophize the whys, maybes, and why-nots of a situation, and then decide to move forward. Deconstructing a conundrum is high entertainment. We see it on political talk shows every day: "*Oui, mais* ..." ("Yes, but...") is how individuals agree with one another.

Still, I never cease to be intrigued and impressed by the process. Intellectual gymnastics are a competitive sport in France. Conversation is an art, one that all Frenchwomen have mastered.

Generally speaking, the French are a highly imaginative and visionary people whose lives often reflect a seamless cohabitation with the past, present, and future. That's what makes them so interesting. At the same time, they wish to protect the best of their *patrimoine* (cultural heritage) while inventing totally modern innovations, be they in food and clothing or fiber optics and high-speed trains.

When decorating their homes, for example, there is nothing Frenchwomen like better than giving a nod to the past by allowing an inherited Louis XVI commode to keep company with an Eero Saarinen Tulip table and Philippe Starck Ghost chairs. Why not?

Patrimoine is also a precious element of French family life. As a young widow, Carol Duval-Leroy took on the responsibilities of the outstanding Champagne house of the same name. "It's our name on the Duval-Leroy bottle, so it's our reputation," she says. "Our reputation is precious." She is now working with her adult sons. Her young grandchildren, who sometimes scamper around her office while she is working, will be the seventh generation to carry on the family tradition. Duval-Leroy Champagne is an integral component of the family's history and, as I discovered while sipping their Champagne with Carol and her sons, it is most definitely part of their everyday *art de vivre*.

LES BONNES MANIÈRES

Often when searching for a simple definition of good manners, the word "kindness" comes up. That, of course, is the foundation of politesse and civility. For example, at the end of my lunch with Carol Duval-Leroy, she said to me, "Who can I call to help you with your book?"

She then called Pierre Hermé, the famous pâtissier, whose name is synonymous with arguably the world's best macarons; Philippe Gombert, the president of the Relais & Châteaux group; and Éric Fréchon, the Michelin three-star chef of Le Hôtel Bristol in Paris. Her calls were the introduction that gave me immediate entry into my interviews with them. Sometimes I think that the natural reserve that the French often display is misinterpreted as being standoffish or unfriendly. In my long experience, I have been spoiled with kindness.

Les bonnes manières is also a choice: a choice to present oneself in a certain way, with the understanding that our comportment must be impeccable—appearance is nothing if our personality displays rudeness, arrogance, or disrespect.

To delve more deeply into the role of good manners in *l'art de vivre,* I turned to an expert and spent an afternoon drinking tea at the Hôtel Lancaster in Paris with Albane de Maigret, a highly respected authority on *les bonnes manières* past and present—and, she dearly hopes, the future. Our conversation was absolutely captivating. She described *l'art de vivre* as a particularly French sense of historical significance that permeates life.

"We are steeped in our history, and as a result we tend to have certain values that have persisted," she says. "Good manners and gallantry—although I regret we're seeing less gallantry—make life infinitely more agreeable."

A few days later I met with Stéphane Bern for coffee. For years, he has been one of my absolute favorite Frenchmen, even though we had never crossed paths. Thanks to my friend Françoise Dumas, mission accomplished. I kept hoping I wouldn't be disappointed.

I wasn't.

Stéphane Bern is the host of the enthralling French television program *Secrets d'Histoire* and a veritable encyclopedic reference for *l'art de vivre,* protocol, royalty, and *les bonnes manières*. He has been inducted into the Order of Arts and Letters in France, the Order of Grimaldi in Monaco, and the Order of the British Empire (the OBE).

As an expert on French history and protocol in several countries, he is a scintillating interview and a coveted invitee at the best parties in Paris. In fact, when some hosts and hostesses are not entirely sure about certain obscure protocol procedures, whether it's the number of shots in a gun salute according to the guest of honor's rank or an honored guest's placement at table, they call him. Having Stéphane at the table is a great coup for a dinner party.

Back in the day, it was said that ambitious hostesses would invite the Duke and Duchess of Windsor, who lived in Paris, to soirées to bolster their reputations and then send a piece of jewelry, mutually agreed upon, to the Duchess, thus sealing the deal. When the invitation was officially accepted, the hostess built her guest list around the presence of the couple and voilà, she moved up another rung on the ladder to social success.

A lucky hostess could most definitely build a dinner party around Stéphane Bern.

As I was saying, when I posed the questions, How do you define *l'art de vivre à la française?* Stéphane's response was perfect: "*L'art de vivre à la française* is a link in a chain of refinement and elegance. While in a sense it is codified, at the same time it adapts to the demands and requirements of every situation."

"Good manners, *savoir faire*, courtesy, and respect are not constraints. On the contrary, they become part of a comfortable behavior that is ultimately liberating. Knowing how to act in all situations is a form of freedom."

The French understand we can slightly adjust our comportment to myriad circumstances while remaining ever in the context of politesse and respect. The codification of madame, monsieur, and mademoiselle on first meetings and then following the everyday "*bonjour*" and "*au revoir*" exchanges in boutiques and for acquaintances is a perfect reflection of a social code that makes life easier. From the very youngest age, children are taught that a "bonjour" must always be followed by the appropriate form of address: "Bonjour, madame; au revoir, monsieur."

What if you momentarily forget someone's name? Madame, monsieur, and mademoiselle solve the problem, no name required. Unfortunately, Americans don't have that fallback.

QUALITY: FROM THE SIMPLE TO THE SUBLIME

Another detail we must never forget in this broad discussion of *l'art de vivre*: quality.

Quality is defined as "the standard of something as measured against other things of a similar kind; the degree of excellence of something." The definition can easily apply to the intangible—think impeccable manners and consideration for others—and to things that can make our lives more attractive and fun.

Seeking quality, however one interprets it—a single gold bangle; huge, old linen napkins from one's great-grandmother or the flea market; an heirloom crystal vase; a Chanel jacket; a grandmother's needlepoint evening bag; masses of garden flowers in a simple clay pot; a four-ply cashmere throw; a thoughtfully crafted handwritten note on lovely paper—is a way to enrich one's life. Frenchwomen of a certain age know that when they surround themselves with beauty, contentment follows naturally.

We are, after all, the curators of our lives; we can always choose the lovely over the banal.

We are, after all, the curators of our lives; we can always choose the lovely over the banal.

Quality, the best of the best, is so revered in France that special awards have been established to honor those who have produced remarkable excellence in their given field. One such decoration, established nearly one hundred years ago, is the *Meilleurs Ouvriers de France* (MOF) medal, which honors the finest craftsmen and -women in the country. The award for special abilities is unique in the world. Today, along with classic cherished métiers of the past that still exist, new, more modern trades and high-tech fields have been added to the list of professions. The MOF is given to the best producers of everything from cheese and pastries to glassmakers and silversmiths to textile designers and jewelry artisans. Each category awards three medals: gold, silver, and bronze. The Camembert in our refrigerator and the crunchy sea salt–infused butter in the butter dish both boast gold medals.

THEN THERE IS HARMONY

All is right with the world when our lives are in perfect harmony, notwithstanding the annoying way life can sometimes disrupt the smooth flow of contentment and serenity. Still, my friends and almost everyone I interviewed talked about the importance of harmony for a life well lived.

From Gilles Odin, director of one of France's major nurseries, and Philippe Gombert, president of Relais & Châteaux, to the renowned Michelin three-star chef Michel Guérard, harmony was the leitmotif that ran through almost everyone's definition of *l'art de vivre*.

"I recommend walking in a forest," Gilles Odin says. "Appreciating nature is an essential part of *l'art de vivre*."

One of my close friends, Chantal, takes her three dogs into the Rambouillet forest every day "for at least two hours," she says.

Both my artist friend Edith and my French niece take long walks in the forest and fields near our houses after Sunday lunches. It matters not at all to them if it's raining, snowing, hot, or cold. Nothing stops them. They dress accordingly.

Philippe Gombert says he sees harmony "in all that surrounds us—a *potager,* a table setting, a bouquet, a perfectly ripe fruit. Think about the guiding principles to which the members of Relais & Châteaux adhere. I think they perfectly define *l'art de vivre à la française*: calm, courtesy, charm, cuisine, and character. I believe they are excellent goals to apply in one's life, don't you?"

Yes, I do.

"Remember, too," he adds, "our heritage is very dear to us, and we protect certain aspects of our past, among them rituals that are important for a certain quality of living. UNESCO, for example, has protected our gastronomic patrimony."

In 2010, UNESCO declared that France's multicourse gastronomic repast—with its attendant rites and presentation—fulfilled the requirements to be included on the revered "world intangible heritage" list. The list seeks to protect cultural practices in the same way UNESCO is dedicated to protecting sites of cultural value or great natural beauty. France's ambassador to UNESCO at the time, Catherine Colonna, noted that the French enjoy getting together "to eat well and drink well. How wines are paired with dishes, how the table is dressed, the precise placement of glasses for water, red and white wines, and the fork tines down are all seen as part of the rite," she says.

(Also protected under UNESCO are France's Alençon lace making, Aubusson tapestry, traditional dances of Brittany, and equitation "in the French tradition." I'm rather surprised that haute couture and the arts and crafts that embellish its creations have not been included as part of France's intangible heritage. Perhaps they will be one day.)

The ambassador's eat-well-and-drink-well aside was, not surprisingly, mentioned by almost everyone I met. I would definitely add that to my definition of the *l'art de vivre* question.

In separate conversations with Michel and Christine Guérard, he one of the world's most celebrated chefs and she greatly admired for her exquisite taste and refinement, harmony is the couple's way of explaining *l'art de vivre à la française.*

"Try to be happy every day," he says. "Consciously celebrate the positive rapport we can have with one another; never be in conflict. Always search for harmony."

"I do not want to live my life in a sad way," Christine Guérard says. "The world is difficult, we see that all around us, but I believe in being a romantic. I decorate our homes and our hotels to evoke a feeling of romanticism. The idea of harmony mingled with audacity is very appealing to me. I've tried to maintain the wonder I had as a child. I was immersed in fairy tales and have never forgotten the joy they gave me. I try to transmit that feeling in whatever I do."

Both Monsieur and Madame Guérard have been awarded the prestigious Ordre National de la Légion d'Honneur (National Order of the Legion of Honor), established in 1802 by Napoléon Bonaparte, originally as a military honor but later to reward merit in several domains.

Jean-André Charial, owner of Baumanière les Baux-de-Provence and the Michelin two-star chef of its restaurant, L'Oustau de Baumanière, and his wife, Geneviève, have created a little corner of paradise in Provence and both deeply appreciate their good fortune.

"Everything here is a reflection of *l'art de vivre* and *joie de vivre,*" he says. "I believe in the 'force' of a place. Every day I look at the light. I walk through my *potager,* the olive grove, and breathe in the air and the calm. Geneviève and I are surrounded by beauty everywhere we look."

For her part, Geneviève talks about the "magic" of their environment: part nature, part self-made by the artistic eye she takes to decorating the rooms and suites. And again, she speaks of harmony. "For me, harmony is the most important goal in life. It's in the cuisine, the decoration of the dining rooms, the hotel rooms, and the suites, the way we speak, the way we present ourselves."

Interior designer Jahel Gourdon describes *l'art de vivre* as "the sensation of comfort one feels in *chaleureuse* [warm] surroundings, a good meal, and a good wine.

"It's also an ambience that the French look for when choosing a restaurant," she adds. "We like a warm, encompassing ambience, an atypical place, calming music."

A REVERENCE FOR WORDS

Le mot juste, the precise word to express oneself in a situation, is almost a parlor game in France. The search for the perfect word is the extension of the French adoration for lively conversation. Time and again in my interviews, observers of outstanding French hostesses say they are the masters of *le mot juste* and sparkling conversation. It's part of their reputation; it's why everyone wants to be invited to their parties, I was told. The majority of these hostesses are *les femmes d'un certain âge.*

With their passion for words and language, it is only logical that the French, and Frenchwomen of a certain age in particular, love and celebrate books. France's rich, revered literary past and present are intrinsic components of *l'art de vivre*.

There are two highly respected television programs that discuss the latest releases, often by theme, which leads to animated exchanges. Apart from international prizes, inside the country there are five major prizes for literature. The most coveted award is the Prix Goncourt, followed by the Grand 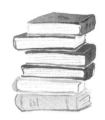 Prix du Roman de l'Academie Française, Prix Renaudot, Prix Femina, Prix Médicis, and Prix Interallié, as Marie Dabadie, the Secrétaire Générale of the Académie Goncourt, shared with me when I had the pleasure of sitting next to her on a recent flight from Paris to Bordeaux.

"The Prix Goncourt results in a minimum of 300,000 book sales," Marie tells me, noting that a recent winner sold more than 800,000 copies of her book. "It was a great book," she adds. I've always known about the French passion for literature, but I had no idea that apart from the top five, there is another layer of approximately 1,200 awards writers can receive.

I have rarely been to a French dinner party where someone doesn't begin a conversation by talking about what he or she is reading, particularly in the autumn when the season's highly anticipated books are released.

Marie confirmed what I had heard. Women are the principal buyers, consumers, and givers of books. "The statistics tell us that the largest group of women is between thirty and fifty years old," she says. "We love to read books, and then we pass them along to friends with our recommendations explaining why we think they too will love the book we just finished." At the moment, she is giving her friends the historical novel and winner of the 2017 Goncourt Prize *L'Ordre du Jour* by Éric Vuillard, which she told me would be "absolutely" worth the effort it would take me to read it in French.

My French niece, who not long ago celebrated her fiftieth birthday, tends to read two books at the same time, one fiction, the other nonfiction. Books as gifts are coveted, and it's rare that the giver has not read the book she offers a friend so that she can explain why she liked it.

"When in doubt, give a book," is the motto of most of my friends. A book is one of those gifts that can be given to that friend who has everything. When it comes to books, no one has everything.

STYLE AND CHARM

An essential part of *l'art de vivre* revolves around personal style and charm, something Frenchwomen of a certain age are renowned for. To be considered charming in France is one of the most appreciated compliments a woman (or a man like Stéphane Bern, for example) can receive. It's that difficult to explain but easily recognizable sparkle that enchants anyone who enters into the person's magical orbit. Jacqueline de Ribes, Doris Brynner, Terry de Gunzburg, and Mathilde Favier are irresistible. Each one in her own definitively individual way is chicly elegant, but it's their charming allure that sets them apart.

My wonderful friend Françoise Dumas spends her life surrounded by some of the most stylish and charming women in France.

Françoise and her business partner, Anne Roustang, are responsible for creating the most glamorous parties in Paris and Monaco. Their clients include Karl Lagerfeld, Chanel, Bernard Arnault, and the coterie of brands under the LVMH label from Dior and Givenchy to Guerlain and Château d'Yquem Sauternes. They have produced special dinners at the Élysée Palace, soirées for famous Paris hostesses like Countess de Ribes, and exceptional celebrations for the royal family of Monaco and various dignitaries.

Recently, she and Anne conjured up a sumptuous evening at the Grand Palais in Paris to celebrate the opening of "Joyaux des Grand Moghols aux Maharajahs," an exhibition of 270 extraordinary Indian jewels.

With chandeliers over the huge table, the backdrop of the museum, the flowers by Eric Chauvin, the food by Michel Guérard, and the exquisite *art de table*, the result was breathtaking, even for jaded international partygoers.

I met the ever generous Françoise more than thirty years ago when I was working as a contributing editor on fashion and lifestyle for the *International Herald Tribune,* the Paris correspondent for the *Chicago Tribune,* and acting editor of *Elle.* (It's amazing what one can do when one is young...) I am forever grateful to her for helping me as I tried to navigate my way in the *haut monde*

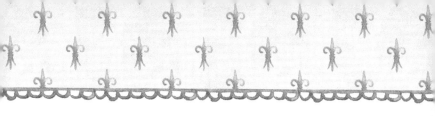

A Living
LANGUAGE

I find that protecting a country's language is a remarkable expression of its *patrimoine*. The preeminent Académie Française, founded in 1635 by Armand-Jean du Plessis de Richelieu, the Cardinal Richelieu and King Louis XIII's First Minister, is the supreme example of France's intrinsic respect for words. The revered forty-member body of intellectuals elected to the Académie for life watch over all matters regarding the French language.

And yet reverence for language does not preclude yearly additions to the lexicon that enrich its vocabulary. With a tweak of pronunciation, the literal invention of new words, the addition of accent punctuation, and sometimes changes in spelling, the pages in the dictionary grow annually. Here are some recent additions I thought you might find amusing:

UBÉRISER: not an Uber-user, but a new—and some French people worry about this—way the globalization of *métiers* are becoming individualized. Airbnb falls into this growing category.

TWITTOSPHÉRE: the world of twitter.

AQUABIKE: the bicycles in swimming pools for exercise. Where I swim you have to sign up at least a day in advance to use them and if you are two minutes late to the pool, you lose your place. They're *very* popular.

RELATIONNISTE; someone in charge of public relations, although it sounds more like someone in charge of one's mental health.

ÉCOCITÉ: areas or neighborhoods that respect the environment.

ÉMOJI: you know what that means.

FABLAB: no, this is not a fabulous laboratory—it's a laboratory that makes things, i.e. fabricates.

AMBIANCER: to add ambiance to an event.

GEEKER: someone who spends an inordinate amount of time in front of a computer.

SPOILER: just like in English—don't tell me how the book ends, don't tell me the denouement of my favorite TV series.

TROLLER: again, as in English, people who write nasty material on social media, usually anonymously.

YOUTUBER: just as it sounds, but to add a certain French *je ne sais quoi*, in its feminine form, it becomes *youtubereuse*.

ZÉNITUDE, my favorite, a feminine noun that loosely translates as that moment of total serenity and calm one hopes to attain right in the middle of a yoga session.

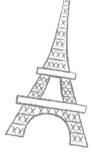

of sophisticated Parisian parties when my French vocabulary consisted of ten to twenty words that were never assembled into a sentence with a verb. When I interviewed her for this book, she opened her little black book so that I could easily contact some of the best hostesses and style icons in France.

"Here is Mathilde's telephone number, you *must* call her," she said. So I did.

Mathilde Favier, VIP public relations director for Dior, is a member of the ultrachic and minuscule group of insiders often referred to as Les Parisiennes—capital L, capital P—indicating that she is head-turning stylish, with a sparkling intelligence and glorious smile that makes her one of those women who is often photographed out and about in Paris, New York, Los Angeles, and beyond.

She is absolutely divine: gamine, exuberant, blade-of-grass thin, effortlessly chic, kind, and, in short: fun to be around. She is the very essence of charm. She lights up a room.

"*L'art de vivre* is about refinement, paying attention to details, charm . . . it's about giving and paying attention to others," Mathilde says.

"When I'm planning a dinner party, for example, I always think: What will make my guests happy; what do they like to eat? I think it's important to try to please people. It's a great pleasure to set a pretty table. We were raised to understand the importance of making our dining tables and our homes pleasing."

She looks at dressing in the same way: it should be fun every day, and why shouldn't looking at the way women turn themselves out be a form of entertainment for others?

After our first meeting, drinking tea and eating macarons in her gorgeous Paris apartment with her dog, Muesli, sitting on my lap, I noticed she was wearing three fine-chained necklaces of graduating lengths. When I arrived home, I took out my necklaces. I haven't worn necklaces in years. I'm more of a bracelet-and-earrings sort of accessorizer. Shortly thereafter, to my great surprise and pleasure, I received a new necklace for my birthday. Now I'm layering necklaces, too.

Next, Françoise Dumas said to me, "You *must* interview Doris Brynner, she is wonderful. You'll love her."

I did and I do. She is also a great friend of Mathilde's.

Doris Brynner was, until recently, the director of the Dior Maison boutique, where she imbued the once painfully classic emporium with her celebrated reputation for impeccable taste, creativity, and audacity. Former French culture minister Frédéric Mitterrand once referred to her as a "symbol of chic." That she is.

She was awarded the Order of Arts and Letters, which is further testament to her vaunted reputation.

She thinks the best way to interpret an appealing *art de vivre* is "to live the best way you can within your means, wherever you are."

This advice comes from a woman who was once married to Yul Brynner; was best friends with Audrey Hepburn, who was her daughter's godmother; and has spent her life in some of the most glamorous places in the world, with some of the most glamorous and interesting people in the world.

When you meet her, you wish she were your best friend. Doris Brynner is warm, straightforward, and immensely kind. I felt exceptionally fortunate have spent time with her.

"*L'art de vivre* has nothing to do with luxury or money," she says. "It's a way of treating everyone in the same way, of making people feel comfortable. I cannot stand chichi. It's important to be relaxed, to not be stiff and artificial."

Often, the word *simple* is an inadequate adjective because it can seem either disingenuous or not sufficiently well understood in its use as the most sincere compliment. When Doris uses it, you understand its value.

"I love simplicity in all aspects of our lives, from the home to clothes," she says. "I never follow fashion, I don't see the point in it. It's more interesting to adapt to our style and lifestyle. After a certain age, we know this, I think."

Unlike many fashionable women in Paris, Doris Brynner loves color. The day we met for tea, she was wearing a bright green coat. She was the single spark of color in a restaurant overflowing with women in various interpretations of black, me being one of them. It was delightful to see her break the mold.

A few weeks later, I saw her at a magnificent party—arranged by Françoise and Anne—and hosted by Jacqueline de Ribes at a benefit for the Musée d'Orsay in Paris. That evening, Doris was wearing a mauve-and-deep amethyst ensemble. She spent much of the event surrounded by women, and lots of men, who wanted to greet her.

A few days before that evening, Françoise had invited me to a divine soirée at the Château Mouton Rothschild because, as she said: "I think you'll enjoy the evening, and I think it will help you with your book."

Once again, she was right. One of my heroines was at the dinner: the head-turning stunner Christine Lagarde, managing director of the International Monetary Fund.

I drank my flute of Champagne for courage, stood at the end of the line of her admirers, waited my turn, and blurted out that I am a Christine Lagarde groupie (totally true), and if it would not be too impolite on my part, could I please ask her two quick questions for the book I was writing.

She thanked me, assured me I was not being impolite, although I probably was, and said, "Meet me by my table after dinner."

I asked her to please tell me her definition of *l'art de vivre à la française*. "It's a combination of elegance, dignity, and irony," she says. "Irony is very important."

You'll find her answer to my second question in Chapter 6 on style and dressing. If you are familiar with her striking style, you understand why.

The very glamorous and the very beautiful Terry de Gunzburg, mother of four, grandmother of ten, is famous for the iconic makeup products she created as the artistic director of Yves Saint Laurent's beauty line. When you think of Touche Èclat, think of Terry. Every other makeup brand in the world has. If Coco Chanel was right that imitation is the highest form of flattery, then Terry is spoiled in that regard. She has had her own line of luxe cosmetics, By Terry, since 1998, coveted by those in the know. She also has a reputation for being one of Paris's and London's most remarkable hostesses.

Over tea and strawberries in her lovely Paris home, we discussed everything from beauty to dinner parties and, of course, the subject at hand. (I would not be exaggerating in the slightest by telling you that literally I drank gallons of tea during the preparation of this book.)

"Removing all vanity from one's life is a way to be happy," she says. "I think it's essential to be attached to sentiments, not things, and I think it's useless to be disagreeable."

She wholeheartedly believes makeup—"not a lot"— is another component of *l'art de vivre*. (See Chapter 5: Beauty for more on this.)

Throughout the reign of the French kings, the women inside and outside the court used makeup to communicate their intentions and signal their social positions. Today, makeup still speaks volumes about us and how we wish to be perceived. The subtle use of cosmetics enhances a woman's beauty and communicates her confidence—*l'art de vivre* indeed.

FINDING THE INSPIRATION

My wonderful Francophile friend Marsi constantly reminds me that information becomes more valuable when it's "actionable." It's true that *l'art de vivre à la française* is part philosophy, but at the same time it's also *intent*—in other words, we can assimilate aspects that appeal to us to assemble our own definition of *l'art de vivre.* Here is how I translate the idea into action for myself:

- A French-inspired "inspiration board" covers one wall in my office. On it are photographs, pages from magazines, quotes in French, an outfit I find inspiring, images of bouquets, ideas for table settings, French-inspired postcards from friends, invitations to parties like the one from Jacqueline de Ribes to the Friends of the Musée d'Orsay dinner illustrated with Paul Cézanne's *Boy With a Red Vest,* and so on.

- Lavender batons woven with pretty silk ribbons are scattered on all the shelves of our linen closet. Embroidered sachets are in my lingerie drawers. I refill them every year using the lavender growing in our garden. I even make my own potpourri (more on that in *Un Cadeau,* page 230).

- One shelf in my kitchen has only French cookbooks. My best French friend, Anne-Françoise, gave me a cookbook as a wedding present. It was my first volume. It not only helped me learn how to prepare a few classic recipes, but also added to my vocabulary and helped me learn more about the metric system.

- I've taught myself how to cook a handful of simple, no-fail recipes. All my *entrées* (starters) are on the table when guests sit down. It makes entertaining much easier. Anne-Françoise taught me that trick as well. Our dinner parties are very French in the sense that they are course by course, or *à la française.* (More on that in Chapter 4: Entertaining.)

- I have a file folder with dividers into which I have assembled recipes, table-setting ideas, articles on wine, bouquets, and menu recommendations. I add to it and refer to it often.

- I have subscriptions to French decorating magazines: *Côté Ouest, Côté Sud, Côté Paris,* and *Elle Décoration.* I have also maintained my subscription to French *Elle* magazine. It's a weekly, which is exciting, and usually I learn something useful. My husband accuses me, not without reason, of whipping through the pages at a speed that does not justify the investment in the prices of the subscriptions. What he doesn't realize is that the ideas fly off the pages, and I rip them out to place in my file folders or pin to my inspiration board.

- Regularly I try to read books about French life and history, usually translated into English because although I can read in French, my mastery is more compatible with newspapers, magazines, and the internet. History and novels are difficult and very time-consuming for me, which takes away the pleasure, I'm sorry to say.

- Even after all these years, I make it a point to learn a new word or two every day. I have a very rich vocabulary that is unfortunately not the case with my verb tenses.

- I follow the French lead and save certain foods and recipes for the fall and winter, and others for the spring and summer. In fact, to my regret, it's almost impossible to buy a fresh-scooped ice cream cone in the winter in Paris.

- I dress the part. In other words, I make the effort each

day. As I sit here typing this chapter, I'm wearing black trousers; a black, long-sleeve T-shirt; a taupe zip-up cardigan "borrowed" from my husband; a large taupe scarf with tiny black polka dots; black ballet flats; a tinted moisturizer; brows cleverly enhanced with an eyebrow pencil because I have never really been blessed with what one could legitimately call "eyebrows"; hair in a ponytail; and perfume. If I need to leave the house later in the day, I'll add my favorite slightly tinted lip gloss and my prescription sunglasses, which double as eye makeup.

FINAL THOUGHTS

L'art de vivre and all it entails is not a facade. It is a multifaceted philosophy of life. No one understands this better than my husband, or as I have referred to him for years in my blog, My-Reason-For-Living-In-France.

THIS IS WHAT HE TOLD ME: "It's the faculty of *émerveillement* (wonder) that is right there for all of us if we're open to it. Let's say you're unhappy for some reason—go outside, listen to the birds, observe the light, look at the dew on the grass, breathe deeply, look at the love in the eyes of your dog.

"Develop the faculty to admire and appreciate simple pleasures. We can fabricate happiness even where others might not see it. It's important to learn how to observe—really observe—and be open to experiences, to envelop ourselves in our imagination."

You see? I learn something every day.

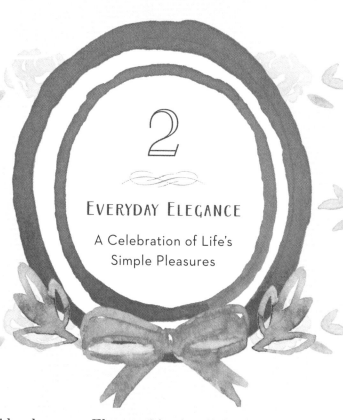

2

EVERYDAY ELEGANCE

A Celebration of Life's
Simple Pleasures

Ah, elegance. Elegance is simplicity in its purest form, expressing grace, refinement, and a certain charm. It is about the way we look, but also the way we act. Elegance is at the heart of *l'art de vivre à la française*, which is why it merits a more in-depth exploration including how, specifically, we can incorporate elegance into our daily lives.

THE ROLE OF POLITESSE

Whenever the subject of elegance arose in my interviews, the first thing universally mentioned was impeccable behavior in all circumstances. Politesse and elegance are inextricably intertwined. A woman can have closets full of haute couture; own homes around the world decorated by instantly recognizable names; and order her bouquets from famous florists and her food from renowned caterers. But if that very same woman lacks decorum, treats others with disdain, holds court, speaks loudly, shows no interest in another's conversation, interrupts, or doesn't listen when someone speaks while she mentally prepares her clever response, she is not elegant.

One of my absolute favorite explanations of politesse is from Germaine de Staël, the revered eighteenth-century writer; daughter of Jacques Necker, Louis XVI's finance minister; and assembler of one of Paris's most extraordinary salons. She declared that "Politeness is the art of choosing among your thoughts."

> "Politeness is the art of choosing among your thoughts."
> —GERMAINE DE STAËL

Imagine if we actually spoke some of our thoughts. Most of us would alienate family members and have few friends. Discretion, kindness, and civility are censors for errant unkind thoughts that might enter into one's mind. Madame de Staël built her stellar reputation on her intelligence, wit, and masterly refined conversation. I could go on and on about her because I've read the remarkable biography, *Madame de Staël: The First Modern Woman,* by Francine du Plessix Gray, which I highly recommend.

The exquisitely well-mannered Terry de Gunzburg, the creator of the luxury cosmetic and perfume line By Terry, says that she tries every day "to be a better person. Not perfect, you understand, just better. I'm very respectful of people who work in any form of service. I hate spoiled people who treat others badly. The more spoiled I am, and I am spoiled in so many ways, the more I am emotionally removed from vanity. I know how to live in the moment. I understand that everything can disappear in an instant. It is totally useless to be disagreeable. I process bad behavior and walk away. I will not dispense energy on toxic people. I want to project and surround myself with positive energy," she says. You see—elegance inside and out.

ELEGANCE IS A GIFT

I have the distinct impression that my French girl-friends and acquaintances, many of whom are grandmothers now, see passing along lessons for everyday elegance and politesse as a way of giving their families an invaluable gift.

From the youngest ages, French boys and girls are instructed in *les formules de politesse.* I remember decades ago being invited for dinners *chez* Anne-Françoise and Daniel, and their six children, including the youngest, who at the time were four and five, stood when adults entered a room and greeted us with "Bonjour, madame" and "Bonjour, monsieur." (Sometimes they needed a little coaching, which I always found adorable.)

The idea, of course, is that good manners become reflexes and, as we all know, it takes diligent repetition to assimilate a reflex. While it's true that there are certain codified rituals of behavior in France, almost everyone agrees that once learned—and that means consistent repetition when children are very young—habit sets in and good manners and respect follow naturally. Call it nagging, call it harassment, but at the end of the day, we're giving the gift that keeps on giving for the rest of their lives. Although it may take hundreds of boring repetitions to instill the natural reflex of good manners into a child's behavior, it's worth it.

"It's not so much standards of comportment that I wanted my children and grandchildren to learn," Anne-Françoise tells me. "It's simply the most civilized and pleasant way to live one's life. I wanted my children and now my grandchildren to understand the importance of good manners and the small, everyday rituals that make our lives more pleasing."

At a recent Christmas celebration, Anne-Françoise and Daniel and their entire family—twenty-six children, grandchildren, and cousins—gathered for "an exceptional fete," she says. "It's rare these days when we are all together, so it was truly *superbe*." When I peppered her with questions about the weeklong reunion, she gave me some of the details: "Yes, of course, everyone dressed for Christmas Eve dinner, you know me. We spent a great deal of time at the table, there was much gaiety, and everyone was on their best behavior," she says.

Albane de Maigret, an expert and professor of *savoir vivre*—literally "know how to live," but understood in French as kindness, tact, and *les bonnes manières*—

emphasizes the importance of always treating one's family with politesse. "Good manners with our families are a mark of respect and affection," she says. "I've never understood those who fall into a *laissez-aller* comportment with those closest to them. Standards of behavior are important."

Savoir vivre is a way of living well with intelligence and enjoyment by meeting every situation with poise and good manners, as Albane de Maigret points out, while *savoir faire* (to know or to know how to do something) is the confidence and ability it takes to act appropriately in social situations. Together, these form the foundation for everyday elegance, whether *en famille* or in public.

ELEGANCE INSIDE AND OUT

"Elegance is when the inside is as beautiful as the outside," Coco Chanel once declared. Now, before you think that

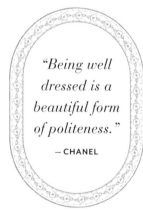

"Being well dressed is a beautiful form of politeness."

— CHANEL

elegance is artifice or in any way superficial, it is anything but mere facade. Our way of dressing reflects our intentions and our attitude. It's a way of hinting at the inside out. This goes for our homes, too. A well-decorated home is essential to an elegant life. Our homes should give us a familiar frisson of well-being when we walk through the front door. Our homes are another reflection of who we are, and the details within its walls should be important to our contentment.

Frenchwomen of a certain age are truly the standard-bearers of elegance. They learned it from watching their mothers and grandmothers, and now that they have taken over those roles, their children and grandchildren are picking up the mantle. I see how they set the standards in all aspects of their lives, not only in the way they decorate their homes, but also in how they maintain them. The latter means running a household that functions without stress and mess and with a warm, welcoming atmosphere.

Nonchalant elegance is a hallmark of Frenchwomen—at least that is the impression they like to project in most aspects of their lives. It seems somehow innate, and for some, I suspect it is. It most definitely seems to be a natural part of the busy life of Dior's Mathilde Favier.

"What is elegance?" she ponders. "It's never pretending to be someone you're not. It's trying to figure out who you are and stay true to who you are and take advantage of that strength. Never speak too loudly, listen—always listen—and stay humble. Don't ever think it's all about clothes or appearances. It never is. Dress for the occasion. Have a positive attitude, and take it with you wherever you are and with whomever you are interacting. Pay attention to your posture; it speaks volumes. And always, always be well-mannered." She adds, "My mother is very elegant, and she made everything look easy."

With Mathilde's glamorous life working and socializing with her A-list friends and clients, her access to some of the most exquisite clothes in the world, and her placement at some of the best parties in Paris and beyond, one might think that she would be, well, spoiled for lack of a better word. She is not. She is warm, kind, and delightfully unpretentious. She truly lives by her definition of elegance. She returns telephone calls immediately, answers e-mails quickly, and is ever polite, which is not always the case with some of her peers in Paris, particularly in the business of fashion.

The delightful Camille Miceli, creative director of jewelry for Louis Vuitton, is one of Mathilde's very best friends, and it's easy to understand why the two are practically inseparable. They positively radiate elegance and *joie de vivre*; both smile all the time. They appear not to have a care in the world, and the aura they project is infectious.

Camille defines everyday elegance as "the art of generosity, distributing kind gestures throughout the day, and that definitely includes our families," she says. "I got up at 6:00 a.m. this morning to make a special breakfast for my son because he had an important exam, and I wanted to make sure that he was OK—mostly because I just like being with him. Now I'm a bit tired, but happy."

In our morning meeting, we admired the small arrangement of pinky-coral carnations tightly packed into a small cylindrical vase in the center of the table where we were having our coffee. For some reason, the arrangement started a conversation about peonies, which we discovered are our favorite flowers.

"Did you know that peonies love to be caressed?" she asks me. No, I had no idea. She then explains that stroking them ever so gently makes them happy and more beautiful. Isn't that sweet? I think the gesture is yet another example of everyday elegance.

All of us can "stroke" others with kind gestures and words and watch the happy result. I can actually see the expression on my dog's face change when I tell her how much I love her and stroke her head. The possibilities for spreading joy are infinite.

I have never met Venezuelan-born designer Carolina Herrera, but I have seen her walking down the street in New York City. Her elegance is crisp and her grooming irreproachable. It is quite different from the more nonchalant elegance one tends to associate with Frenchwomen, which is to say that elegance comes in many forms, but it's easy to recognize when we see it. It's an outward expression of personality.

I mention Carolina Herrera because I found her definition of elegance to be pertinent and interesting: "Elegance is not only what you're wearing, it is how you wear it, who you are *inside*. It is the way you decorate your house, what you surround yourself with, what books you read, and what your interests are," she says.

YOU SEE?: It permeates all facets of our lives, and we can choose to live with elegance. It *is* a choice: a choice about the way we present ourselves and our homes; how we maintain relationships with friends and family members; and how we exhibit respect in everyday encounters with people we may never see again. These are the inner and outer manifestations of true elegance. Simple, *non*?

"MODESTY, WHAT ELEGANCE!"

Elegance is often defined as refined grace and dignified propriety. Dior's Mathilde Favier says she thought it was important to add humility to her definition: "We must always, always remain humble."

Modesty in dress and comportment are elegant. As Coco Chanel said, "Adornment, what a science; beauty, what a weapon; modesty, what elegance!" How in the world did we get to the point where the most vulgar and narcissistic behavior has become popular entertainment or, worse, an aspirational goal. Elegance is not self-importance, snobbery, vulgarity, or arrogance.

TIME FOR A DISCLAIMER: I suspect we can all agree that a flash of leg, an almost backless dress, and some cleavage—assuming that these constitute some of a woman's best assets—displayed at the appropriate times and places can be most attractive. But I have never seen a Frenchwoman expose herself on all fronts. Indecent exposure is not her thing. She believes in the allure of the imagination.

Young women love their very short skirts from time to time, and why shouldn't they? Women of a certain age with lovely legs wear their skirts above the knee, and good for them. Others prefer a skirt that hits just below the knee—whatever works. Here's the thing, though: Frenchwomen, and particularly those of a certain age, love *mystery*. A hint of beautiful lingerie might peek out of a sober jacket, but it's just a little tease. How seductive is that?

Their definition of sexy is often an esprit presented in a demure package, which might or might not be unwrapped. Overexposure is rarely their modus operandi. From what I've witnessed during my three decades in France, the often flirty rapport between men and women is not merely, or not necessarily, a game of physical seduction; rather, it is often a game of intellectual seduction. In some circles, it's a national sport.

While we're on the subject of questionable comportment, let's not forget about bad behavior, sometimes aggressively so, which seems to be a socially acceptable part of the international scene. We read about it, observe it, see it in the media, watch it on reality-TV series, and then forget about it. It becomes stimuli overload, and our discerning systems shut down.

For many, profanity has become popular verb and adjective choices. Rarely have I heard my French friends or acquaintances use profanity. As I said, they are setting examples. They prefer *le mot juste*. Imagine the impact of the perfect word spoken at the perfect moment.

Lying, too, has become the new normal. My-Reason-For-Living-In-France and I sat in front of the television watching the French presidential debates, wherein blatant lies were flying from the glossed lips of one candidate toward the other. It was startling. But the most unsettling moment was after the debate, when the candidate flaunting the untruths looked into a flock of television cameras and accused the other of lying. It was astonishing. I asked my husband if I had somehow misunderstood the French. He assured me I had not. On that front, it appears that no country has a monopoly on untruths.

"It can be disheartening to see the multiplication of incivility in today's society," Albane de Maigret says. She also laments a certain *laissez-aller* in our quotidian. "It is not because we are with our families that we should fall into negligence and disrespect. Respect and *savior faire* are essential components in a civilized life," she says.

While on the subject of questionable behavior, I knew a woman in New York, a member by marriage of one of America's great families, who was, in shocking ways, snobbish and rude. She was very kind to me, but whenever I was with her in public, I often felt embarrassed and uncomfortable. She was curt with waiters, condescending with doormen, and snappish with salespeople. And yet when she was with her friends, her manners were beyond reproach.

> *"We must never confuse elegance with snobbery."*
> — YVES SAINT LAURENT

She was an extraordinary hostess, set a lovely table, served delicious meals, and listened to her guests without interruption. She was cultured and well-read, she spoke fluent French and German, and classical music and opera played in her apartment throughout the day. She possessed a formal library with hundreds of leather-bound books, all of which she had read. She had closets filled with designer frocks and boxes of gasp-worthy jewelry. The missing element was elegance.

I think we all agree that those whose job it is to serve us in any capacity merit our utmost respect. A career dedicated to dealing with a difficult public cannot be fun.

True elegance is not a concept that can be turned on or off depending upon situations or even one's mood. It is a way of *being*. It's that *savoir faire* again. Above all, it is synonymous with grace, poise, and consideration for others.

ELEGANCE AT THE TABLE

My daughter refers to my granddaughter's visits to our house in France as "Ella's finishing school." At age three, she learned to say, "May I please be excused?" before leaving the dinner table. She had already been bombarded—on both sides of the Atlantic—with her *please*s and *thank-you*s. It was so sweet to see her run from the table, remember, run back, half sit down, and ask if she could be excused. One day it will become a reflex, and then if she too has children, she will remind them to please ask to be excused from the table.

Some gestures of good manners are logical; it's simply rude to abruptly leave the table. Other expressions of politesse have interesting historical raisons d'être.

"All matters of politesse have explanations, and some anecdotes make for interesting conversation," Albane de Maigret tells me. She then recounts what has now become one of my favorite stories: the explanation for why dinner knives have rounded blades. Their invention dates back to the extremely refined and elegant Cardinal Armand Jean

HOW DO WE
define ourselves?

Life is full of challenges. It can be messy—literally and figuratively—and a solid dose of good behavior can help us deal more calmly with inevitable obstacles. Here is a little checklist on how to adapt and deal with unpleasant people and circumstances:

- Ask yourself, Who am I? How do I want to be perceived? How do I want my behavior to transmit my definition of me?

- Losing control of one's temper, arguing with cruel rebukes, and engaging in emotional blackmail are neither kind nor elegant. Composure is. Think grace under pressure, then breathe deeply.

- Ostentation is the inverse of elegance. According to Coco Chanel, "Modesty is the highest elegance."

- Speak clearly, explain respectfully, and listen. It's not always necessary to be right. Sometimes being gracious is far more effective.

- Learn how to say no with pleasant firmness. Declining to do something that one does not wish to do, for whatever reason, is a trait Frenchwomen have perfected.

- Making promises you will resent keeping is a miserable idea.

- If your comportment is a true reflection of the principles that define you, then you never have to waste time worrying about what other people think about you.

- Pick up a pen and write an occasional note. We all know the utter joy we feel when we see that special envelope in our mail.

du Plessis, 1st Duke of Richelieu and Fronsac (1585–1642), who was appalled by one of the distasteful uses of the very pointed knives that were an omnipresent accessory of men in that epoch. Their knives were an all-purpose tool for hunting, dining, fingernail tidying, and—what the cardinal could no longer tolerate—picking and cleaning teeth at the table. Even though the cardinal was an exceedingly busy man, not only as Louis XIII's most prominent minister but also, as I mentioned previously, as the founder of the Académie Française, he still decided he needed to act on the knife issue.

One can definitely sympathize with his sentiments. And thus our rounded knives were designed to Cardinal Richelieu's specifications in an effort to make dining experiences more civilized by eliminating the distasteful utility of a pointed blade.

While we're on the subject of cutlery, let me talk about setting an everyday table for the family. Why shouldn't the table be pretty? It's not complicated, and it adds a touch of elegance to the routine. Everyone will appreciate the slight effort involved.

French interior designer Jahel Gourdon sets a pretty dinner table every night for her family. "I like to vary the plates, place mats, glasses, and flatware," she says. "We always have a small round or square vase on the table with *petites fleurs* and a sprig of greenery."

One of my close friends, a widow, always sets a pretty table for herself. If you'll pardon the marketing line from a famous cosmetic brand, she likes to say, "Because I'm worth it."

While visiting my family in the United States, I interviewed Sébastien Canonne, cofounder of the French Pastry School in Chicago. Apart from discussing—and eating—pastry, the adorable Sébastien, who was awarded the *Meilleurs Ouvriers de France* (MOF), the French Ministry's highest honor for craftsmen, told me about one of the mealtime rules in his home. "The dinner table is the one place where everyone can talk about their day, and if you happen to have children or grandchildren, it can be the moment when they let something slip that will give you some insight into what is going on in their lives," he says. "It's also a time to appreciate good food at the table with family. Healthy, interesting food presented attractively is a way to teach children from the very youngest age to appreciate and enjoy not only the food, but also the experiences shared at the table. Good food and good conversation go together."

A WORD ABOUT MODERN CONVENIENCES: All electronics should be silenced and placed in another room before sitting at the table. Why is a telephone more interesting than the people with whom one is dining? Parents and grandparents who check and respond to messages on their cell phones while with their children or grandchildren are signaling that they are not interested in being with them. Children pick up on the vibe and the priorities. Instead, let the conversation begin.

EVERYDAY LUXURIES

Frenchwomen know the value of taking a creative approach to the everyday, the mix of the utilitarian with the luxurious and the basic with the beautiful. Truly, the devil is *always* in the details, particularly the small, often unexpected ideas that make the everyday special. Inspiration is everywhere if we pay attention (or ask lots and lots of questions ...).

Elegant seems to be an appropriate adjective to describe Sylvaine Delacourte's creations from her time at *chez* Guerlain and in her new eponymous collection. Each of her fragrances has a distinct personality, rich with nuances and unexpected finishes. She even has simple, unexpected ideas on how to use perfume. One of her favorite ways involves making a rainy day more pleasant.

"I spray the inside of my umbrella with perfume," she says. "I love the idea of a one-note rose, for example. Then when it rains, you feel like rose petals are falling on you. It changes *everything* on a dreary, gray day." It does indeed. I used a lavender eau de cologne I often spray on my sheets and pillowcases inside my umbrella, and it made me smile. It was a lovely surprise.

When it comes to simplicity and elegance for the home, arguably no one has translated the notion more perfectly than the inimitable Doris Brynner, the woman responsible for making the Dior Maison collections uniquely covetable. She proved that humble materials—wicker accessories and olive-wood flatware—can be simply elegant and unspeakably chic table accessories.

"I'm against *argenterie* [silverware]," she declares, somewhat ironically I suspect. "I love glassware—vases,

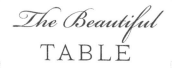

The Beautiful TABLE

Here are a few simple ways to make your table more pleasant:

1. Dressing the Table Pretty place mats make meals more appealing. They tend to be easier than a tablecloth for everyday use.

2. Use Cloth It's not difficult to find no-iron napkins and save the extra-large ones that need to be ironed for more formal dinners, unless you have someone who does your ironing or it is a chore you enjoy.

3. Keep it Informal Christine Guérard, who is responsible for the exquisite decoration for the Les Prés d'Eugénie hotel, restaurant, and spa, takes a large napkin, picks it up in the center, and places it unfolded on the table. The effect seems like a nonchalant accessory tossed to the left of the plates. "Starched, ironed, and perfectly folded napkins are too labor-intensive," she says. "I also like the look of a napkin casually draped on the table."

4. Decorative Details Find an appealing center decoration, anything from a single flower or a plant to a bowl of pine cones or a platter of fruit or an objet d'art. On a terrace table with linen runners, Christine Guérard places three lemons in the center of the table, but you can use whatever is on hand. Be inventive.

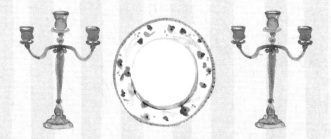

5. Play with Color My friend Françoise Dumas, who arranges some of the world's most glamorous parties, tells me that in her vacation home in Portugal, she often uses colorful glasses she finds at local markets or from Monoprix when she entertains. "Pretty is pretty," she says. "Everything doesn't have to be expensive." (Monoprix is one of my absolute favorite stores. It's sort of like a very French, very stylish version of Target.)

6. The Warmth of Candlelight In the winter, candles lift the spirits. They can be particularly pretty inside hurricane lamps, which can be left on the table as permanent decorations.

7. Presentation is Paramount No cartons or boxes of anything on the table, *ever*. Water in a pitcher or a simple carafe, milk in a pitcher for breakfast. Pizza is on a platter or served in the kitchen buffet-style and brought to the table on a plate. The only bottle containing a liquid that is to be poured into a glass would be wine.

8. Why wouldn't You? All beverages for the entire family at the table should be consumed out of a glass.

beautiful drinking glasses, plates, sometimes hand-painted. They can add wonderful color to the everyday. I like color. I like it at the table; I like it in clothes," she says. "Wicker I'm absolutely mad about. It's charming, simple, elegant."

Often she will give one of her wicker objects as a gift to friends. Some of the items are practical, like Pyrex serving pieces that slip into the chic camouflage of wicker for presentation on the table. Others have a sober elegance, like her wicker trays. I would love to have one of her trays for garden entertaining. She, however, uses wicker for year-round entertaining in her Paris apartment.

Doris likes the mix of the practical with the pretty, the high with the low. She has built her stellar reputation on her ability to pull off that harmonious cohabitation with great flair.

Flowers are another way to add elegance to your everyday life. I adore flowers and can't imagine living 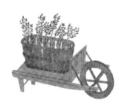 without them in our house. When I look for inspiration for bouquets I visit one of my favorite "secret" addresses in Paris, Catherine Muller's flower school. If it were possible, I would visit her every week to stock up on the most exquisite flowers I have ever seen gathered in one place at the same time.

Walking through the door of her Parisian flower school is like entering a magical world of utter beauty, not only for the take-your-breath-away fragrance, but also for the masses and masses of seasonal flowers. In buckets and tubs of water, the unarranged blooms, branches, berries, leaves, and other offerings from nature spill out onto the sidewalk in front of her tiny emporium. And here's the thing: nothing is for sale. Every element is an ingredient waiting for her flower-arranging classes.

It is possible to buy her beautiful candles, each created by her and faithfully replicating single-note fragrances of some of her favorite flowers. They are presented in a cylindrical box with a silk ribbon corresponding to the color of the flower within. Other items one can buy include tools to facilitate bouquet construction and linen garden aprons and smocks. But not a bouquet or even a single bloom can be purchased. It's frustrating.

"I teach other florists and interior designers, and it wouldn't be professional if I were competing with them," she says.

Her four-day workshops have themes like Provence, Marie Antoinette, retro style, and weddings and are open to anyone interested in learning how to make beautiful arrangements. She also has schools in London and New York City.

One of my very best friends, the Francophile, author, and renowned interior designer Betty Lou Phillips, told me I should meet Catherine. How right she was. I even sat in on one of Catherine's lessons and came home with a massive bouquet I couldn't believe I was capable of making. It was an unforgettable experience, and I am very grateful.

Catherine is perfectly capable of turning out intricate constructions, which she did for former clients such as Cartier, LVMH, Dior, Céline, the Palais Garnier, Jane Birkin, and Catherine Deneuve, but she tends to prefer the simple over the sophisticated. "Mother Nature does things much better than we do," she says. "Nature is varied enough that you don't need artifice."

She explained how she loves to take armloads of flowers and let them fall as they may in a large container. "It is so pretty to see them settle in comfortably without being arranged," she says. She demonstrated just this in the class I attended to prove her point.

Flowers are intrinsically elegant, and Catherine insists that there is room in every budget for a flower or a bouquet or something gathered in a field or forest. "Sometimes I'll use wheat, bare branches, and berries together or separately," she says. "The rule about flowers is that there are no rules. Really, it's simple. What is more elegant than nature?"

(For Catherine's specific seasonal bouquet ideas, please see *Un Cadeau*, page 237.)

MAKING THE EFFORT

I fully realize that some like to argue elegant living is a dusty relic of the past, and that the small effort it takes is a waste of time. Many aspects of our lives involve a series of choices and decisions. How we deal with them is up to us; my choice will always be making that effort.

Assembling routines that help our lives run smoothly does not preclude streamlining the details to accommodate busy schedules. Routines are also the ultimate time saver once in place. (More on this in the Homemaking chapter.) Everyone is busy these days, no

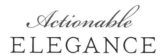

Actionable ELEGANCE

I think it's time for more everyday-elegance pointers from Albane de Maigret that, once again, make the quotidian more pleasant:

- When entering a restaurant in France, the man enters first to "open" the path for his companion. When a couple is led to the table by a waiter or a maître d'hôtel, the woman takes the lead.

- When a restaurant has a banquette, it is given to women. In any case, the seat facing out toward the restaurant is reserved for the woman.

- Absolutely no makeup repair is to be conducted at the table, and that includes whipping out a compact to reapply lipstick.

- Always offer a "bonjour" and an "au revoir" upon entering and leaving boutiques and doctors' waiting rooms.

- When calling someone's home, after "Hello," give your name, followed by "May I please speak to . . . "

- Never call during the hours that are considered mealtimes, like 12:00 p.m. to 1:30 p.m. and 7:00 p.m. (meal preparation) to 9:00-ish.

- When confronted with an unpleasant service situation, try to be calm and not escalate the exchange.

- A wonderful friend of mine passed on a lesson she learned as a mother of four. "We must never tell friends about the normal, everyday discipline problems we may have with our children. Friends will remember forever, and we will have long forgotten. Just like with our partners, we owe our children respect," she says.

question about it. Still, if *easy* is construed to mean "Who cares?" what a shame that is.

Surely there is something uplifting and peaceful about surrounding ourselves with simple elegance, feathering our nests with the things that make our homes a spiritually safe and beautifully restorative haven.

A subject that has caused surprising debate on my blog is dressing with care as opposed to "Who cares?" I recounted a story about meeting a woman for an interview at an elegant Parisian hotel (for tea, what else?) and being taken aback when I saw her disheveled appearance. It wasn't precisely what she was wearing, it was the wrinkled, unkempt nature of her clothes and scuffed shoes. And yes, I did make that assessment in less than ten seconds.

Some readers chastised me for my shallowness and asked me whether I left the interview with useful information—I did. Absolutely, it was her choice to present herself as she did, but I couldn't help but wonder why she didn't wish to represent her brand with an image that silently spoke for her before she said a word.

In my desire to be kind, respectful, and open-minded, I've tried to understand why someone wouldn't use her or his appearance as a simple means to communicate a positive message. Whatever one's decision in that regard, a *communiqué* is being sent, and the interlocutor is the interpreter.

"Dressing for occasions is another form of elegance and respect," Albane de Maigret says. Mathilde Favier concurs, adding that "dressing up is so much fun."

I agree. Maybe I will never understand why some women have decided that polishing their appearance is of no importance to them or that dressing up is a chore. I am willing to wager that all of us enjoy seeing stylish women. One of my favorite pastimes is sitting in a Parisian café with a *café au lait* or a glass of wine watching Frenchwomen of all ages parade before me in their varied expressions of vestment creativity. It's theater at its best.

I am a huge proponent of taking joy where we can find it, and I believe grooming and creative dressing guarantee major returns on time invested. Why, then, would we deprive ourselves of that satisfaction? Making the effort to look the best we can is one of the most positive, morale-boosting gestures we can do for ourselves. It reflects respect for ourselves and others. It is everyday elegance before a word has been spoken.

A LIFE WELL LIVED

Beyond the exterior expression of elegance—the way a woman applies her makeup, arranges her hair, dresses, decorates her home, and entertains, and the books she reads, her passions, and her interests—at its core, elegance is the reflection of the interior: poise, politesse, and purpose. It's part of the refinement and rigor that encompasses a life well lived every day.

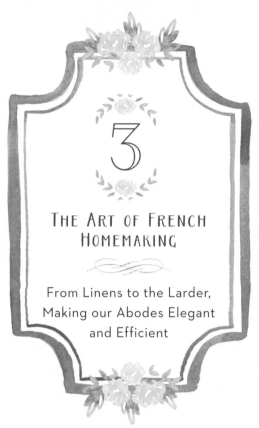

3

THE ART OF FRENCH HOMEMAKING

From Linens to the Larder,
Making our Abodes Elegant
and Efficient

Frenchwomen take the idea of caring for their homes very seriously. As with all of us, they have chores they enjoy, like ironing and silver polishing, for example, and others they like less well, but all of my friends and acquaintances maintain lovely homes because it makes them happy to live in beautiful, ordered environments.

In a conversation with Christine Guérard, who is responsible for the sumptuous decoration and the smooth running of Les Prés d'Eugénie hotel, spa, and restaurant with her husband, Michelin three-star chef Michel Guérard, she told me how excited she was about her latest project,

Académie des Gens de Maison, a school that will teach the art of housekeeping. The classes will include everything from flower arranging and bed making to ironing and setting a proper table, among other household skills.

Madame Guérard is a proponent of efficacy and elegance, which she believes are the keys to a beautiful home. Her original idea was to only train hospitality professionals, but she realized that her academy would also be of great interest to the public. I'm hoping to sit in on some of the classes. Imagine what one could learn in her academy and apply to one's abode.

Like many aspects of the quotidian, I discovered that when it comes to homemaking, I could learn a great deal from Frenchwomen, particularly those of a certain age, because they have fine-tuned the tasks to near perfection over the decades.

My friends have told me that they keep order, beauty, and convenience in their homes by ensuring that their closets—both linen and clothes—are intelligently and attractively organized in ways that allow instant no-fuss access to what they need. At the same time, they offer a delight for the senses in that they are sweetly aromatic and aesthetically arranged so when the doors are opened, every day they are pleased by what they see and inhale.

Frenchwomen's organizational techniques continue to the kitchen. They learned long ago that a well-stocked larder is indispensable for a smooth-running household. Being prepared for the everyday and the unexpected seems to be their mantra.

Several of my friends—namely Chantal and my artist pal, Edith (if you read my last book, you met her in the wardrobe chapter where I told you how she wore an ankle-skimming fuchsia cotton skirt in scores of iterations)—are majorly into doing their part for the planet, so their cleaning products are minimal and ecologically friendly. My wonderful *femme de ménage* (cleaning lady or housekeeper), Elise, uses only natural products. She has taught me a great deal about conscientious cleaning.

For Frenchwomen of a certain age, keeping house is a combination of art, science, and tradition. Decorating, cooking, and entertaining are the art. Science comes in with the cleaning, maintaining, and organizing. Finally, tradition is the special ingredient that each family brings to the whole by adding its unique mix of culture, heritage, and customs.

> *When all the components are in harmony, a household runs smoothly and pleasantly while providing a restorative retreat for all within.*

In the following pages, I move through the house examining every detail. I consulted a few very old French books owned by my husband's mother and grandmother for help and, as always, my friends and experts for tips on the fine art of homemaking à *la française*. The old books are so much fun and demonstrate the inventiveness of women over the generations, long before store-bought cleaning products became big business. For example, the notion that the water from boiled potatoes makes a great starch for shirts and sheets is intriguing (though not intriguing enough for me to try it).

THE FRENCH LINEN CLOSET

Let's begin with linens.

Frenchwomen take very good care of their linens. Delphine Beltran, the artistic director of D. Porthault, referred to by those in the know as purveyors of *haute couture linge de maison*, explained that by treating bed, bath, and table linens properly and in some cases delicately, they can be passed on for generations.

In many cases, bed and table linens have been in families for generations and using them preserves and celebrates a familial history.

A collection of lovely linens is a treasure. It includes the crisp, sweetly perfumed sheets we slip into after a bath, the pillows scented with lavender to help us sleep better, and the towels that smell like springtime. Then there are the napkins, the tablecloths, and the place mats that make the everyday prettier and entertaining more elegant.

I wanted to learn more about buying, collecting, mixing and matching, and caring for beautiful linens, so I turned to Delphine for her expert advice.

When I asked her about the idea of linens being passed down through the generations in French families, she says she has always appreciated the symbol they represent. "Bed linens are particularly personal and intimate, and there is something quite marvelous about keeping them for a very long time," she says.

"All linens, including tablecloths and napkins that remind children and grandchildren of their family history, are yet another way to communicate. Each item can remind us of memories of lunches in the country, holiday celebrations, or our best friend sleeping in a bed dressed with our grandmother's trousseau sheets and pillowcases."

Delphine also likes the idea of mixing the old with the new.

"I like the audacity of the mélange of epochs," she explains. "It's fun and creative to revive the past with a more modern universe of colors, prints, embroidery, or lace, for example. It's a way to revive our patrimony and, of course, every time we combine the new with the old, we're adding our personal touch, our own history, if you will."

Next, I thought it was important to have her opinion on what one should have in her linen closet. (I specified "after a certain age" to see if I was covered on that front.) As it turns out, Delphine very much considers bed and bath linens as an opportunity to use our decorating skills.

"Really, there are no rules," she opines, adding that she finds it elegant and desirable to be able to coordinate bed and bath linens "the way we do in our collections. It's much like dressing in a way—the foundation and the accessories coordinated to enhance the effect."

She continues, "It's lovely to have sets of sheets and changeable accessories so that one's bed can be arranged according to one's mood. Percale is an excellent choice for its *fraîcheur* (freshness); the silky feel of cotton sateen and the sensuality and softness of cotton voile offer different but pleasing elegance and comfort."

D. Porthault is known for its sophisticated prints, introduced into the world of bedding at the debut of the twentieth century when everyone was "sleeping on traditional white and ivory linen," according to Delphine. Also added to the palette were dressmaker details, some of which remain in the Porthault archives and are repeated in current collections, while others are newly inspired.

"The mix of the different universes of color and prints or white with trim produce an atmosphere that expresses one's personality," Delphine says. "The bed can be the center of a room's decoration, and it can be changed constantly. Having that liberty—to mix and match or stay pure to white on white with or without trim—is certainly another vision of luxury and elegance."

If you do not own D. Porthault towels or bedding, you may have experienced the exquisite pleasure of their comfort and beauty if you have stayed at the Hôtel Ritz, Hôtel Bristol, Hôtel Meurice, Hôtel de Crillon, or the Plaza Athénée in Paris; the Pierre Hotel in New York; or Relais & Châteaux properties throughout Europe.

Clearly, high-quality household linens can involve considerable expense when purchased new, but they are a multigenerational investment that will be well worth the initial cost. Every time I use a tablecloth and napkins that belonged to my parents, I think of them. What a lovely way to be remembered, don't you think?

If budgets do not permit, flea markets, particularly those in France, present a satisfying alternative. I have never been to one where I haven't seen stands stacked high with all varieties of household linens—everything from napkins and dish towels to tablecloths and bedding—at very affordable prices. Plus, you can usually negotiate.

I've found many linen dish towels at flea markets, and in one of my favorite places deep in the country west of Paris, I met a woman who dyes old linen sheets and tablecloths the most luscious, soft colors. I bought a large pale, watery blue linen sheet and another in a barely there mauve, both of which I use as tablecloths.

Like my French friends, I keep sachets of lavender in my linen closet and lingerie drawers. Some I buy, others I make from the lavender in our garden. I have a collection of small sachets in cotton, tulle, and floral fabrics from Provence that I tie with silk ribbons, and when the fragrance disappears, as it inevitably does, I simply refill them. Just because they are so very pretty, I slip in *bâtons de lavande*, the stems and blossoms of lavender woven together with silk or velvet ribbons. (There are tutorials on the internet on how to make them, if you feel so inclined.) These are the tiny luxuries that do make a difference in your home.

I like the way my friend Anne-Françoise color-coordinates her linen closet because, as in so many of the ways she organizes her household items from linens to china to glassware, she brings her artistic touch to her collections even behind closed doors. My linen organization is not complicated but still pretty, I think: all of my towels are white, some have colored borders, and more color comes in with my sachets and lavender *bâtons*.

My sheets are the same, white with detailing, which is sometimes white on white or a single color embroidery. We do have two sets of lusciously extravagant and absolutely beautiful sheets from D. Porthault. One is white sprinkled with a field of faded blue flowers, the other is the palest pink. They are at least forty-five years old and have a softness I cannot describe after probably hundreds of washings.

We also have a few sets of white linen sheets that have been in my husband's family for generations, each one with intricate embroidery embellishments. They are lovely, soft to the touch while cool to the body as you slip between them on a hot summer night. There is something irresistibly soothing about tucking into a bed with linen sheets. However, linen involves considerably more work, so they are used less often as a consequence. Making a bed with wrinkled sheets is extremely unappealing, and ironing them is a major project. Still, each time I see them in our linen closet, they are so pretty that just a glance gives me pleasure. When layered over a plump dining-table pad, they can be extremely elegant, and I tend to use them more in that context than on our beds.

Like my French girlfriends use it, color may enter into the exterior "dressing up" of beds: on *boutis* (quilts), duvet slipcovers, pillows of all sorts, or a cashmere, merino, or mohair throw placed on the end of the bed. *Boutis* also double as divine tablecloths.

I canvased a few of my friends, Anne-Françoise (of course), Jeanne-Aelia, and Chantal, about how they stock their linen closets—how many sheets for each bed and any other tricks they might like to add. This is what they told me:

- All agree that three sets of sheets for each bed would be the minimum, while at the same time noting that they have several linen sets passed down from their mothers and grandmothers that they use less often even though they are a dream to sleep upon—ironing them requires more dedication, so they tend to save them for family reunions and guest rooms.

- For Anne-Françoise, who has a huge family and entertains often (guests sometimes visit for a week), the three-set rule applies to her guest rooms. She names her bedrooms and has affixed the names on the front of the shelves to correspond to each room, such as *Papillon* (Butterfly). Towels for the en suite bathrooms are color-coordinated with and next to the sheets. In this way, she is ever ready for visitors. For her own bedroom, she has many more sheets and bedding accessories because she likes to change the look quite often, she says.

- After laundering bed and bath linens, the newly clean items go on the bottom of the piles to guarantee rotation to extend the life of the fabrics.

- My friends recommend six to nine pillowcases to accompany the three sets of sheets, because they never make up a bed with only one pillow.

- *Boutis* abound in their households because they like to change the mood in their bedrooms.

❧ Decades ago, Anne-Françoise stopped ironing her sheets from top to bottom. "I just iron enough on the top so that when I turn the sheet over the blanket, it looks pretty. Who is looking under the bedcoverings?" (I was sure she ironed every centimeter. She's just like the rest of us.)

❧ They empty and clean out their linen closets once a year. The cleaning includes removing the paper covering the shelves, dusting, washing down the shelves and sides with *savon de Marseilles* (the internationally renowned soap made from Mediterranean olive oil and volcanic ash), and adding new papers and sachets. We all love Marseilles soap because its cleaning capabilities are unmatched, it has been used for centuries (which gives it a certain historical caché), and it is completely biodegradable.

❧ Jeanne-Aelia folds her bottom fitted sheets into the ironed top sheets before arranging the set in her linen closet. "That way, the bedding for each room comes out together," she says. "I only choose white sheets," she adds. "I love cotton sateen and bamboo fabrics the most. I definitely change the bed coverings depending upon the season: different decorative pillows, duvet covers, and throws. Always lighter colors in the spring and summer and darker, richer, warmer colors in the fall and winter."

FRENCH HOUSEKEEPING SECRETS

I am lucky to have a lovely *femme de ménage,* Elise, who uses primarily old, tried-and-true, and, may I add, 100 percent biodegradable products when cleaning. She has taught me a great deal over the years. She gives me a monthly list of items for her cleaning needs, and I stock up. These are some of our favorites:

- Liquid *savon de Marseilles* for the laundry. It's pure and fresh. Bedding and towels smell like they've been dried on the line in a beautiful garden. We have a beautiful garden, but I use our dryer most of the time.

- *Savon noir en pâte* (black soap paste), works wonders for cleaning ovens, stove fans, and metal garden furniture. When diluted in warm water, it is an excellent antiseptic shampoo for dogs. It's also a great substitute for purpose-made silver-polish products. Dilute four tablespoons in warm water, plunge silver in the liquid, wait five minutes, remove, rinse, and polish with a soft cotton cloth. *Savon noir,* black soap, made from olive oil, is, like *savon de Marseilles,* totally biodegradable and cleans everything (including our bodies). For centuries black soap has been used in hammam baths to cleanse and exfoliate the skin. I've tried it in a hammam and it's a divine experience.

- White vinegar for windows and the inside of the refrigerator. It makes chrome and stainless steel shine.

- Fresh lemons, sliced and placed in a bowl with water to clean the microwave. Two minutes does the trick.

A quick wipe down, and all traces of splashed liquids
disappear.

- More lemons to get rid of the deposits from our hard
water inside the coffee maker and the electric hot-
water kettle.

- *Alcool ménager (or household alcohol),* naturally
perfumed with lemon extract (otherwise it has a
disagreeable odor), which Elise pretty much uses for
everything. It's a great anti-grease agent.

- She also loves the products from a century-old family
business, Jacques Briochin. There is something in
the collection that cleans almost everything, and
one performs miracles on windows and glass shower
doors. The one we're using now is *Le Nettoyant
Universel,* or universal cleaner, a pale blue liquid in a
spray bottle.

Just like Frenchwomen, I'm trying to do my part for
the environment, which includes shopping with pretty,
washable cotton and burlap bags to minimize my plastic-bag
accumulation. I often see women out here in the country
where we live doing their daily shopping with a basket held
in the crook of their arm that is filled with baguettes and
has lettuce peeking out over the top.

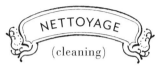

NETTOYAGE
(cleaning)

Here are time-tested tips to take you through the house.

ARGENTERIE (SILVER)

- As I mentioned, we use our silver every day. And do you know what the greatest benefit of this habit is? The silver never needs polishing. Some of our not-often-used serving pieces do, but by using our silver daily, it's so easy to simply polish a few extra pieces as needed.
- For lightly tarnished silver, plunge the pieces in sour milk. Remove from milk after fifteen minutes and polish with a soft cloth.

ÈMAUX (ENAMEL)

Soak the object in warm soapy water, and rinse with the juice of a fresh lemon diluted in warm water.

ODEURS (ODORS)

- When vacuuming, put a handful of potpourri or cloves in the sack. This works well when you live with animals. (You know, the four-footed kind.)
- French interior designer Jahel Gourdon puts several drops of essential oils into the sack of her vacuum. "Essential oils also kill mites," she says.
- To rid the kitchen of unsavory odors without just covering them up, boil a small pan of vinegar for a few minutes.
- A twist on a theme for a pleasant fragrance in the

house: boil a handful of cinnamon sticks and a few cloves; let simmer. It's less complicated than baking cookies and is calorie-free.

❧ To remove odors from rugs, sprinkle generously with baking soda. Let the powder rest for an hour, then vacuum.

TACHES (SPOTS AND STAINS)

RASPBERRIES: Mix the juice of a fresh lemon with hydrogen peroxide, then rinse. (Test on the fabric first.)

GRASS: Blot and gently rub with alcohol, then wash.

EGG YOLKS: Wash with cold water, soap, and hydrogen peroxide.

RED WINE ON A TABLECLOTH: Pour white wine on the spill, cover with salt, and wait until the red wine is absorbed by the salt. Then rub the spot with white vinegar, rinse in cold water, and launder normally.

LEATHER SHOES: Vaseline will remove water stains. Let the Vaseline penetrate the leather before polishing and buffing.

PATENT LEATHER: Rub with a soft cloth soaked with warm skim milk and fresh lemon juice. I love patent leather, and this truly works.

BOUGIES (CANDLES)

❧ To increase their duration, put a few grains of coarse salt at the bottom of the wick, or put them in the freezer for a few hours. This one is from Anne-Françoise.

❧ To help stop the drips from melting candles, soak the candle overnight in very salty water before the first use.

BOUTEILLES ET CARAFES (BOTTLES AND CARAFES)

- To clean those that contained oil, add moist coffee grounds, shake, and rinse. This is easy for me, because I drink French-press coffee every morning and therefore have lots of coffee grounds.

- To clean decorative bottles and carafes, including crystal, combine coarse sea salt with white vinegar and shake, shake, shake. Rinse several times. Distilled water works best as a final rinse.

- For crystal objects, add a few drops of ammonia to a mild dishwashing soap and rinse with warm water and white vinegar. A wonderful friend of mine started giving me Baccarat animals every year for Christmas. I now have a menagerie, so I can attest to the efficaciousness of this system. (I fully realize there are less complicated solutions.)

BOUILLOIRE (KETTLE)

- We use an electric kettle to boil water for tea and anything that requires boiling water. Because our water is very hard, it leaves a lime deposit inside the kettle. To remove the white residue inside, slice a lemon into quarters, fill the kettle, and boil once or twice. With a soft, long-handled kitchen brush, brush the inside and rinse abundantly.

- Once I discovered that putting an oyster shell in the bottom of the kettle eliminates the buildup, the problem was greatly reduced.

TASSES (CUPS)

❧ Porcelain cup interiors stained with coffee or tea can be cleaned by soaking them in hot water with bleach and dishwashing liquid.

MIROIRS (MIRRORS)

❧ To eliminate fingerprints from mirrors, or any glass surface, wipe with ammonia on a soft cloth. In other words, spot-clean.

CHEMINÉE (FIREPLACE)

❧ To revive a fire—at least for a few exciting minutes—toss two handfuls of coarse salt onto the embers or, if you save your corks (we do, and I've never known why exactly), throw them in.

❧ The rinds from lemons, oranges, or grapefruits tossed into a fire give off a delightfully fresh fragrance.

BIJOUX EN OR (GOLD JEWELRY)

❧ Rub with a slice of white bread. I know, I know—it does work, though.

MITES (MOTHS)

❧ Nestle sachets of lavender or mint among sweaters.

❧ Place lots of cloves in a bowl or, as on my shelves, a handful of loose cloves scattered here and there among my sweaters.

RÉFRIGÉRATEUR
(REFRIGERATOR—OF COURSE)

❧ The refrigerator should have a serious cleaning twice a month with a mixture of warm water, white vinegar, and baking soda (one heaping teaspoon for seventy ounces of liquid). To disinfect, rinse with bleach and thirty-five ounces of water. Then rinse again. (My French friends are always very approximative with measurements. When I do this, my vinegar-to-water ratio is one-third to two-thirds. Same thing with the bleach rinse.)

❧ If you need to deodorize the refrigerator between cleanings, before going to bed, place a bowl of hot milk mixed with *herbes de Provence* inside. Remove the next morning.

TISSUS (FABRICS)

❧ To avoid shrinkage, soak a cotton or linen garment or tablecloth before its first use in ice-cold salted water for twelve hours. The water should be extremely salty. I asked Elise about the ratios, and she says "at least one cup [of salt], and it won't make any difference if you use more." She says it wouldn't hurt to empty an ice tray or two into the cold water.

While I was luxuriating in the thermal waters, spa treatments, and *cuisine minceur* diet (more on this on page 244 in Un Cadeau) at Les Prés d'Eugénie, I interviewed Cécile Ledru, the director of *La Ferme Thermale* (the thermal spa). Cécile is an aesthetician and works with the luxury Sisley cosmetic line, as well as overseeing the smooth running of the thermal treatments.

Interviews often veer off in unexpected directions. The original idea with Cécile was a conversation about beauty, but as we talked, I told her I was also working on a homemaking chapter and asked her if she had any unconventional ideas on the subject. She did.

"When I was first married, I made my own laundry detergent," she says. "My husband is a chef, and he comes home with the most stubborn stains on his white coat. I finally found a recipe that never failed to remove every spot."

Laundry Detergent

1 Two-thirds of a cup of grated *savon de Marseilles*.

2 A small glass of *cristaux de soude* (soda ash, or washing soda). A small glass, in French, translates to about six tablespoons.

3 Mix the above ingredients with six cups of boiling water.

4 Add 20 drops of an essential oil of your choice. Cécile uses lavender.

GREEN ADVENTURES

We live in the countryside west of Paris, surrounded by the magnificent Rambouillet forest, where most of us try to be ecologically respectful of our surroundings in our gardens as well as in our homes.

We have lots of fruit trees—apricot, pear, three types of apples, two types of cherries, and two types of plums—and a small *potager* with three kinds of tomatoes, cucumbers, lettuce, mint, basil, thyme, coriander, and raspberries. Some of our friends have what I consider enormous *potagers* that keep them stocked with fruits and vegetables throughout the year.

Undeniably, lovely gardens are part of *l'art de vivre à la française.*

In a conversation with one of my favorite people and our major counselor on our rather *sauvage* garden, Gilles Odin, a landscape artist and the director of a branch of Poullain, one of France's most respected nurseries, he waxed philosophical about the satisfaction that comes from working and relaxing in bucolic havens.

"Gardens bring serenity and joy and, like it or not, they require patience, which can teach us to slow down," he says. "Laying out a garden, or even plants and flowers on a terrace, should be a labor of love and not be rushed. Consciously constructing a tranquil place is more inspiring when it is done gradually."

Thanks to my French garden books, Gilles, and my friends, I never stop learning about how to take care of not only outdoor plants and trees, but also those in the house.

Gilles helped me find bushes that produce berries and clusters of flowers to use in bouquets in the depth of winter. He even ordered special yellow peonies for me. I'm not a natural when it comes to nature, so every bit of information helps

THE KITCHEN À LES FRANÇAISES

My prowess in the kitchen has its limits, but at the same time, my skills therein have been some of my greatest successes since moving to France. That's not contradictory, considering where I started. Apart from mastering a few recipes, I've learned some exceptionally important lessons on how to turn around cooking disasters.

One of the best lessons I've learned from my French girlfriends is to stick with what you know how to do well.

My French niece is a superb cook, and when we're invited for dinner *chez elle*, she almost always asks what we would like, and we almost always say either *pot-au-feu* or poached sea bass with her

In France, the entrée is the first course, as you "enter" into a meal.

delectable hollandaise sauce and small, perfect, unpeeled new potatoes. (It's rare in France to see an unpeeled potato on a plate, so that makes me love her even more.)

She and her husband, also a remarkable cook, like preparing French classics that have become effortlessly easy for them, but because they so enjoy their time spent in meal preparations, they love to experiment with new recipes. Sometimes we're invited to enjoy their experiments.

Another key point is that Frenchwomen of a certain age understand that a well-stocked larder is critical to an intelligently organized, low-stress household. Having the components on hand to make a quick, delicious meal is essential.

To discover what some of those components are, I asked my friends what they always have on hand that allows them to whip up a last-minute dinner for the family or drop-in friends when there is nothing in the pantry.

"I always have the ingredients to make a *tarte salée*, pasta, or a good repast with products from Périgord like foie gras," interior designer Jahel Gourdon says. "Potatoes are always in the house, which allows me to quickly make *pommes de terre rissolées* in goose fat." *Pommes de terre rissolées* is translated as hash browns, but they're much, much better than any hash browns I've ever eaten.

Anne-Françoise makes out-of-this-world omelets; she has a brood of chickens, which helps. She also has a small *potager* from which she can pluck lettuce, a couple of tomatoes, and some herbs.

Once when I was visiting her in Provence, she decided we needed a cake for dessert even though she claimed she didn't have the ingredients. She opened her cupboards, found a bag of chestnut flour, and was inspired. She took a couple of her chickens' eggs, added honey (which she always has on hand from the organic farmer not far from her house), threw in a handful of almonds, added milk, poured everything into a baking pan, and we had cake for dessert.

Dans le Jardin
(IN THE GARDEN)

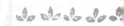

Here are some of my favorite garden
and plant tips:

- I learned that the temperature for the water
used for indoor plants should be the same
temperature as the room. If you have hard water,
add a few drops of vinegar to it.

- Indoor plants love drinking the leftover cooled water from boiled
vegetables or eggs. Supposedly, and Elise says it's true, the water
from boiled potatoes is an excellent fertilizer.

- One of my old books suggested this trick to prolong the life of cut
flowers: cut an X at the base of the stems and dip in olive oil before
putting them in a vase. It works.

- To make a rose bouquet last longer, submerge the stems four
inches deep in boiling water for one minute, then plunge them
immediately into ice-cold water. I always add ice cubes to make
sure the water is *very* cold. We have at least thirty rose bushes,
and they usually continue to bloom well into November and one
mild year, until Christmas.

- To take care of a slug problem (I'm not talking about myself, rather
referring to the slimy ones), try sprinkling coffee grounds on the
soil, suggested by my housekeeper, Elise, or her husband's advice,
small saucers filled with beer. Apparently the slugs get quite drunk
and slither off into the sunset.

- To rid plants of red ants, spiders, and aphids, Elise says, "Mix one-
quarter of a cup of soap in four cups of hot water to 'melt' the soap.
When the liquid cools, pour it into an atomizer and spray plants."

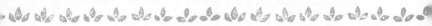

It was my first taste of anything made with chestnut flour. It was delicious, and she served the leftover cake for breakfast.

I think all Frenchwomen always have wine and maybe Champagne on hand. There is also not a French household that does not have long-lasting milk stored in the cupboard or the *cave* (cellar). At this moment, I have six cartons of milk that will be fresh for three months. I *never* run out of milk. Long-lasting milk is not as easy to find in the United States as it is in Europe, but it's worth looking.

No Frenchwoman I know has a kitchen without bread. It's in their freezers as backup—that's where mine is. That means she can serve toast with her omelet. (Most likely she also has a box of melba toasts, just in case.)

Elise makes sauce from the tomatoes and herbs in her huge *potager* and gives us several jars at the end of the summer. Since all types of pasta are a mainstay in our house, a simple meal is always possible.

Another friend, Dany, gives us mushrooms she finds in her secret spots in the Rambouillet forest, which surrounds our village. Some I use immediately—they make a scrumptious omelet or a side dish sautéed in salted butter. Since Dany is generous, I freeze leftovers and add them to Elise's sauce or simply sauté them with the herbs growing on my kitchen windowsill or with fresh garlic and olive oil.

My friend Chantal buys her haricots verts from a local farmer and cans them each fall with her daughter. Her 10-year-old granddaughter recently joined in the family tradition. "An omelet and haricots verts are my instant meal," she says.

I'm not exaggerating when I tell you that every one of my French friends makes her own jams. (Please see *Un Cadeau* page 255 for a wonderful recipe.) They often become gifts for friends. Homemade jam is another one of those presents for the friend who has everything. One year, Anne-Françoise gave me one jar of raspberry jam and another of apricot, plus a bottle of olive oil from their olive trees, all nestled in a small basket lined with a linen dish towel from Provence. I use the basket for bread at the table, and I think of her every time I see it.

Bonne Maman jams and jellies now appear to be available in most countries, and they have attractive jars with their pretty red-and-white Vichy checkered tops to reuse for homemade preserves with your own handwritten label.

Every year when our daughter Andrea visits us in France, one of her childhood friends, Sylvie, gives her honey from her father's beehives. At home in Chicago, Andrea has honey for breakfast and thinks of Sylvie.

Andrea and I started making *bœuf bourguignon*, using the cookbook Anne-Françoise gave me as a wedding present, when she was an adolescent. Today, she makes a large batch in the winter and freezes some of it so that she has it as last-minute backup for impromptu dinner parties. Thanks to Anne-Françoise's thoughtful gift all those years ago, I now have my repertoire of tried-and-true recipes. I've used her cookbook constantly over the decades, and it is starting to disintegrate. I don't want to replace it, though, because every time I open the pages, I think of her.

Finally, while we're still in the kitchen, please do not forget to wear an apron. Almost all of my French friends do, as do I. Putting it on is a gesture that signals a break from one activity to another. Aprons protect our clothes from splashes and accidents, and they are also fun to wear. I categorize them as an accessory and have a little collection.

DÉCORATION

When the good housekeeping rules of organization and routine are firmly in place, it's the decoration of the home that makes it welcoming, chic, and comfortable.

Like Frenchwomen's attitudes toward clothes, one always has the impression that nothing is overly perfect in the decoration of his or her home. Old homes and apartments play to their strengths: high ceilings, original moldings, beams, and creaky parquet floors. Windows are dressed with drapes that puddle elegantly onto the floor. They never skim above the floor, which would have the unfortunate effect of making it appear as if the windows have outgrown their "clothes."

Frenchwomen of a certain age understand intrinsically that the true function of decoration is comfort. Friends who have inherited antique furniture never treat their lovely tables, chests of drawers, or desks as museum pieces. Instead, they mix them in with comfortable sofas, plump with pretty cushions and throws, and inviting wing chairs and ottomans pulled up close to the fireplace. Coffee tables are often piled high with books, a vase of flowers perched on one of the groupings. The feeling is always "home": a reflection of the tastes and interests of a family.

My great friend interior designer Jeanne-Aelia Desparmet-Hart, had the best explanation: "We love the mix of the past and the present in our homes. But, most important, we like the right balance between the perfect and the *à peu prés* (the approximate). I can almost always tell if an interior is French or American. The difference is the inevitable feeling that in the United States everything must be perfectly perfect—level, matching, sometimes over-thought. For us, a portrait with a scratched frame, drapes that are slightly faded, that's fine for us. We like traces of time and history in our surroundings."

The first impression one has when walking into the houses or apartments of my friends and acquaintances is that they are inviting. Anne-Françoise's homes are beautiful without being precious. Dior's Mathilde Favier's sumptuous Paris apartment has been photographed for *Architectural Digest*, but for all its beauty, it is welcoming.

When I asked Jeanne-Aelia for more thoughts on decorating, she not only answered from her point of view, but she also canvased a few friends. "I thought I could give you a more varied picture that way," she says.

"Among the women I know and those I've interviewed in their homes, their decoration has always been lovely and personal. I fully realize that saying all French homes are beautiful is a ridiculous generalization, but this book is about the best of the best, of course," she says with a knowing smile.

Essentials of the
FRENCH LARDER

Frenchwomen always have the
following in their pantry:

RICE

PASTA

FLOUR

CANNED TOMATOES

ONIONS

GARLIC

POTATOES

TOMATO SAUCE

BOUILLON
(chicken, beef, and vegetable)

COARSE SEA
SALT AND WHITE
AND BLACK
PEPPERCORNS

NUTS

HERBS AND SPICES
*(garlic, basil, tarragon,
rosemary, nutmeg, and
bouquet garni, which you can
buy already prepared in little
cheesecloth sacks)*

EGGS

CANNED FISH
*(tuna, herring,
anchovies, and sardines)*

DRIED LEGUMES

DRIED FRUITS

COFFEE, TEA, AND
HERBAL TEAS

"The consensus among my friends is that they love decorating their homes and keep an eye out for what will make them pretty and relaxing. Although each has a very different style, I noticed their home styles were indeed rather similar to their fashion styles and personalities—each liked comfort and practicality. All say a lived–in look is preferred to a magazine-cover one, although most liked checking out decorating magazines and websites.

"Each piece added to a home could be a *coup de coeur*, a makes-my-heart-beat kind of item. In general, my friends would choose the more relaxed piece over the best-looking one. None wanted a complete or a look-at-me home, and each bought what she liked, from wherever and at whatever price, high or low, if it felt right.

"Most thought family items or fond memory pieces were part of the attraction. Acquiring while traveling is a joy for all of them and absolutely essential for me. None followed specific color trends, but those who liked modernism did prefer the midcentury style because it was a trendy look they appreciated."

This reminds me of another friend in Paris who lives in a tiny apartment, furnished from top (literally up to the ceiling with shelves and cabinets) to bottom from IKEA. She then added beautiful embroidered cushions, throws (including an old paisley shawl she found at the flea market), and gorgeous end-of-the-run fabrics from a design house that a friend made into floor-skimming curtains. Her textiles personalize her space and reflect her taste. It's not expensive, yet it's still unbearably chic.

More often than not walls are neutral, and there are scores of neutral colors. (I am married to a French architect, and he is literally obsessed with neutrals.) The background is uncomplicated so it functions as a canvas that can be "dressed" with old mirrors, paintings, photographs, or whatever appeals.

One of my best American friends is a famous interior designer and a Francophile. Many of her clients want French decoration when they commission her for a project. "But the thing is," she tells me, "they want everything to be perfect. They do not want an old armoire to look old, and they do not want to see the patina of age even though they're very clear about requesting furniture that may be museum-quality. Everything must appear new."

In a French home, even those decorated by famous names like Jacques Grange, who helped Dior's Mathilde Favier with her Paris apartment, the first impression when walking through the front door is how beautiful the space is with its white walls, high ceilings, fireplace, mix of vibrant colors against the neutrals, parquet floors, and puddled off-white curtains. Immediately you think, This feels personal, this feels like a home, this feels like a place in which one would be happy and calm. At Mathilde's apartment, you are greeted by her King Charles spaniel, Muesli (she has since added a puppy to her family), and you think, This is definitely a warm, welcoming home. This apartment *is* Mathilde.

Above all, an elegant nonchalance pervades. Throws are tossed on furniture, not neatly folded. Pillows are not

Secrets de Grands-Mères
(GRANDMOTHERS' SECRETS)

These tips come out of an old French book called *Secrets des Grandes-Mères*. Some are familiar, but all are so useful I think they are worth listing:

- **To ripen an avocado,** put it in a paper bag with a banana for twenty-four hours. (My daughter says the same trick works equally well with either an apple or a kiwi.)

- **For more flavor when boiling carrots,** add a teaspoon of baking soda to the water. For even more flavor, add a dollop of crunchy sea-salt butter on top before serving.

- **To avoid the odor from cooking cauliflower,** as well as the slight bitter taste it sometimes has, put a piece of dry white bread in the water, a clean cork (not one from a bottle of wine), or a sugar cube and lemon juice.

- **To avoid gray haricot verts,** sprinkle a pinch of baking soda in the water and cook uncovered.

- **To avoid cracked shells on your boiled eggs,** place a teaspoon in the bottom of the pan and always start with cold water.

- **When a recipe calls for the separation of the yolk and white** and both plop into the bowl, pour the combo into a funnel. The white will go through; the yolk will not.

"broken" with that premeditated karate-chop-in-the-center technique one often sees in non-French homes.

Anne-Françoise has inherited a small warehouse full of beautiful family furniture, and over the years she has passed much of it on to her six children. She has kept some of her favorite pieces that fit into her home and her lifestyle and mixed them in with more comfortable contemporary pieces like cushy sofas and a large glass coffee table.

I don't think I've ever been in a French home without beautiful scented candles placed throughout the house, and one is always on the coffee table. In fact, candles play a major role in the overall ambience, whether scented or unscented.

Music often plays softly in the background. French classic and jazz radio stations have almost no commercials, which makes them an excellent choice for everyday listening. The overall idea is that a happy home is a collection of sensory pleasures.

ON THE SUBJECT OF COLLECTIONS

Collections make a house a home. They are the assemblage of things we are drawn to naturally, and they ultimately bring joy into a home. Some are reminders of precious memories or the continuation of those started long ago by a Frenchwoman's (or Frenchman's) mother or grandmother.

COLLECTIONS ARE A HOME'S ACCESSORIES: Whether consciously or unwittingly constructed, collections reflect our proclivity to surround ourselves with things we love. That's one of the most charming ingredients in making a house a home.

I love baskets. I have a large collection, but it was unintentional. An extra-large one sits next to the fireplace filled with small logs and pine cones to start fires; two in my bathroom hold cosmetics and bath products; one in the kitchen holds cloth napkins; four small ones line the windowsill with pots of herbs—basil, thyme, coriander, mint; and another in the bedroom keeps magazines organized.

Anne-Françoise collects roosters, as in every imaginable image or object thereof, which she has come to deeply regret. They became the go-to gift for friends and family over the decades, and to say she has a flock or a brood would be an enormous understatement. "I try to remember who gave me which one, and when they visit, I take out their rooster, dust it off, and put it on display with the current grouping in the kitchen," she says.

Another lesson learned: Be careful what you wish for.

I collect silver cups, *timbales,* the classic gift given to celebrate newborns in France. Like so many items in our house, the collection was started long before I arrived on the scene. I simply saw it as a marvelous opportunity to keep up a tradition. I had some silver cups with handles, not *timbales,* from my family and over the years I've found others at flea markets. I don't seek them out, but when I find one I like, chances are, I'll try to buy it.

I use them as vases for flowers in water or tiny plants or marching down a table filled with bits of this and that I find in the garden, including herbs.

Two sit on my desk: one holds colored pencils, the other pens, scissors, a ruler, and an antique magnifying glass. Three are lined up in front of the books in our bedroom bookcase, each with a dried hydrangea from our garden.

A couple are on a side table in the dining room filled with bone-handled cheese knives and silver cake forks. A smaller one holds silver and enamel demitasse spoons.

Edith, my artist friend whom I've known for more than thirty years, collects egg cups, and she has no idea how many she owns. Yes, she uses some of them for eggs or in a decorative table grouping, each holding a single blossom or a votive candle, but she also uses a few to mix colors for her paintings.

Terry de Gunzburg collects silver, glassware, and porcelain. In fact, she bought all of Yves Saint Laurent's silver, which is stored in beautiful valise-like cases in her Paris home. Her pantries are filled with exquisite crystal and china, all arranged by set. It's truly breathtaking.

Her collections allow her to do a sit-down dinner, comfortably, for more than 100. If I were to do a dinner for ten, it would be necessary for me to have an ambulance idling in the driveway.

(I don't know whether it's genetic or learned, but I haven't met a Frenchwoman who wasn't calm and comfortable with having large dinner parties. The aplomb they bring to their role as *maîtresse de la maison* never ceases to amaze me.)

I also collect dishes. I get bored with the same plates every day, so I do a lot of rotating and mixing. Even the most banal meal becomes, at least visually, more interesting. Same thing for glasses. We have a marvelous boutique in our village, run by a mother-daughter team that is part florist shop, part housewares. I buy most of my everyday plates, glasses, and colorful bowls from them. Last Christmas, I bought silver water glasses; this year, red.

Several years ago, I started giving Andrea paintings and prints of fruits and vegetables. Some of the paintings are by a French artist, Giles, and others are old prints I have found in Paris and at country flea markets. The quantity has now reached the definition of a collection.

MERCI, MES CHERS AMIS

Over the decades, I have most definitely been influenced by what I've seen in my French friends' homes, from Edith's bohemian vibe and Chantal's country casual (with her three dogs that track in lots of mud, but she doesn't care), to Anne-Françoise's refined elegance and Jeanne-Aelia's French decorating audacity and beauty borne from her mélange of finds collected from living in different countries, including the United States. What they all have in common is an approach to their domestic life that prioritizes organization and preparedness.

They, and the experts I interviewed, set up the solid foundations that make the beauty and mechanics of their homes relatively easy to maintain, so that they may have time to enjoy the fruits of their labors, which is the ultimate *cerise sur le gâteau*—the cherry on the cake.

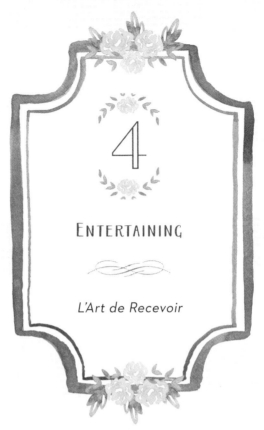

4

ENTERTAINING

L'Art de Recevoir

In France, *entertaining* is translated as *l'art de recevoir*, "the art of receiving," and it is one of the best, and perhaps most enjoyable, ways to celebrate *l'art de vivre à la française.*

"To receive" imparts the sentiment that one is honoring those invited. Whether casual—as in a last-minute phone call announcing that "Daniel is opening a lovely bottle of wine, I'm making an omelet, I just plucked a salad from the *potager,* and we'll find something for dessert, come over right now"—or a month in advance via a calligraphic formal card in the mail, sharing a meal is always an occasion for a celebration. No one knows this better than Frenchwomen of a certain age.

Time and again, the women I interviewed talked about how their mothers and grandmothers influenced the elegance I saw in their homes and the seeming nonchalance they brought to entertaining. As Dior's Mathilde Favier says, "We were raised to understand the importance of making our dining tables and our homes pleasing. When I'm planning a dinner party, for example, I always think, What will make my guests happy? What do they like to eat? I believe it's important to try to please people, to receive with one's heart. It's such a pleasure to set a pretty table.

"My mother always had room at the table for one more person. It was never too late to join us. She made everything seem easy, and she showed us how we could do the same. Thanks to her, my sisters and I love to entertain," she says.

My daughter, Andrea, to my delight, enjoys entertaining and does it quite often despite her busy life. Growing up, she spent an inordinate amount of time at her best French friend Pamela's house. Pamela is one of Anne-Françoise's daughters. Drea was referred to as the family's American cousin.

(Andrea loved to spend time at Pamela's house because it was always full of big family excitement, entertaining, and fun with six children and cousins filling the rooms with bustle and cheer, while Pamela liked to be at our house because it was quiet. From our point of view, neither Andrea nor I, being only children, ever understood the allure of the not-so-much-fun calm in our house.)

Now at home in Chicago, Andrea often chooses to invite friends for Sunday brunch. Children are welcome for brunch, but not when she does "grown-up" dinners. My granddaughter, Ella, clad in her pajamas, says "hello" and "good night" to guests before she disappears for the evening with her babysitter.

When Andrea was in high school, we loved cooking and entertaining together *chez nous*. She is an excellent cook, and most weekends she makes meals in advance for last-minute dinners and impromptu invitations. One of her favorite desserts is an apricot tart, which she claims is fun and "beyond easy." I would like to think that I was somewhat instrumental in her desire to carry on a few French culinary traditions.

My favorite observer of French history and *savoir faire*, Stéphane Bern, had a succinct response for the best recipe for successful entertaining: "The experience should be *bon* and *beau*." In other words, good food enhanced by its pleasing presentation.

This winning combination is not at all complicated and encourages warmth and connection at the table. With that intentional esprit in mind, dinners en famille on a weeknight marking the end of a busy day become part of family tradition.

L'ART DE LA TABLE

From simple everyday dinners or Sunday lunches to more sophisticated affairs, entertaining is part of the rich culture and tradition that comes naturally for the French.

But even for simple everyday entertaining, *l'art de la table* is never neglected. It takes no time to set an attractive table with classic white plates or a mix of different colors and patterns, real napkins, place mats or a tablecloth, and attractive glasses. Pots of herbs can feature in the center of the table, or autumn leaves or whatever is at hand. Each season offers something to appreciate both on our plates and our tables.

The other evening, as I finished putting the dishes into the dishwasher, Alexandra, our niece, called to invite us for lunch the next day. She had just arrived back in Paris after a monthlong vacation while the rest of her family was scheduled to return a week later. Therefore, it was the two of us and Alexandra. She set the table on the tiny terrace of her townhouse with white place mats, red napkins, and blue-and-white plates. In the center of the table, she placed a clay pot with a miniature white rose plant.

For lunch, she made three salads: the first, avocado and shrimp; the second, a classic tomato mozzarella; and the third, a dessert of raspberries and *pêches de vignes*, those sweet, juicy flat peaches. A small basket held pieces of multigrain baguette, and with the post-dessert espressos she brought out a plate with quarter-sized sugar cookies.

All of this she prepared in the morning before she left for her office. She's a doctor. After lunch, she ran to the Metro and returned to her afternoon appointments. She made it all look easy and claimed it was.

When I was staying at Les Prés d'Eugénie, the round iron table on my terrace was set with two taupe linen runners, crossing in the center where Christine Guérard had placed three lemons. It was charming. The rest of the arrangement was pure and simple: white napkin, white plates, unembellished water glasses and wineglasses. The garden provided all the "decoration" necessary, which is exactly the way we feel when we're entertaining in our garden gazebo surrounded by rose bushes, lanterns, and a lovely weeping willow tree that caresses the roof, making the most beautiful sound when a light breeze passes through its leaves.

As Doris Brynner, the mastermind behind the stunning merchandise in the Maison Dior boutiques, says, "Anyone can prepare a good, simple meal and set a pretty table. It's not complicated." She's absolutely correct, but it was a lesson I didn't necessarily learn easily.

In the past, I tended to be an anxious hostess, fretting over every minuscule detail of the menu, wondering whether our friends would enjoy themselves, whether I had timed courses to proceed without an over- or undercooked mishap, and on and on.

I did have one major entertaining disaster not long after our marriage, which was mainly, once again, a misunderstanding of cultural differences on my part. Even Alexandre (my husband) didn't foresee the possibility of the potential misstep when I presented the idea to him.

"Let's do a New Year's Day open house! What do you think?" I proposed with lots of enthusiasm in my delivery.

"Why not?" he responded.

So I sent out the invitations and prepared and prepared

and prepared. As I said, entertaining wasn't a natural reflex for me. Alexandre took care of the Champagne and other wines and put together the cheese choices, while I decorated with a frenzy and filled the dining room with *lots* of food. The idea, as you know, is that people arrive throughout the day, a concept that I should have realized is not part of the French gastronomic lexicon. (It took a couple of decades for brunch to catch on, but now it's quite popular. Who eats a meal at 11 a.m. when lunch will be served at 1 p.m.?) An open house is quite another approach to food that doesn't truly make sense in a country where days are divided into specific times when meals are to be consumed.

Still, our friends were good sports. They came in a steady stream from late morning until early evening, but they ate almost nothing and drank even less. For them, the holidays were over. They had eaten with (relative) abandon in December until the wee hours of January 1, and they were finished. Water, sparkling and still, was the cocktail of choice, and out of politesse, there was a scant amount of crudité nibbling. I considered it remarkably prescient on my part to have included raw vegetables next to the heavier fare. That little catastrophe was a one-off and a lesson learned. The French will indulge just to a certain point and then the payback begins immediately thereafter, in this case on January 1.

Ever since that fateful day, my entertaining has revolved solely around dinner parties.

THE SECRET IS SIMPLICITY

It's always the great chefs and grand hostesses who tell us that the food we serve should be simple, and then they add "and delicious, of course."

RIGHT.

During my interview with Éric Fréchon, the three-star Michelin chef at Le Bristol hotel in Paris, I remarked that I imagined friends would be hesitant to invite him and his wife to dinner in their homes. "*Au contraire*," he said.

His "on the contrary" came with a qualifier: he tells friends, "Make what you know how to do well. Keep everything simple and easy with the best possible ingredients, and relax."

Using the best possible ingredients is the advice every great chef stresses. Never try to make something good that is out of season; it just doesn't work. A tomato salad in December is at best disappointing no matter how outstanding one's recipe for vinaigrette may be.

Fréchon recommends a celery rémoulade in the winter, fresh asparagus with a hollandaise sauce in the spring, and a tomato salad in the summer with a vinaigrette as entrées; a chicken roasted with onions and mushrooms throughout the year as the main course with those delicious little Ratte potatoes all the famous chefs love, slightly softened by boiling, then skinned and sautéed in butter with sea salt. For dessert, he suggests an apple tart with a frangipane crust.

Every Frenchwoman I know can make some version of an apple tart with the greatest of ease, and most of them learned how from their grandmothers—including supervised peeling and cutting of the apples—when they were about eight years old.

"In the summer, a salad of red fruits and vanilla ice cream from Berthillon is perfect," Fréchon adds.

This from a man who says, "I love perfection," and admits that when he has an idea for a new recipe, it can take him ten to fifteen experiments with the ingredients until he is satisfied with the result.

Then, with my new knowledge, I asked him about the cheese-and-white wine combination. "More white wines go with cheese than reds," he confirms. "Though I do like a nice brut cider with Camembert." Some of the wines he likes include 2015 Marcel Lapierre Morgon, a Meursault premier cru, and a Domaine Jamet Côte Rôtie.

ANY WAY YOU LOOK AT IT, learning a few facts about wine, how to perfect a few simple recipes, and how to combine the two is the key to successful entertaining. What would be the point of trying to compete with a Michelin-starred chef?

THE BEST OF THE BEST

Frenchwomen of a certain age have a repertoire of tried-and-true recipes, the ease of which depends upon their culinary talents. I have friends in Paris who know where to shop for the best food from the best caterers. They may (or may not) prepare one course themselves when entertaining and then make certain the bread, cheese, and desserts are scrumptious.

Doris Brynner enjoys entertaining and says that, for her, "cooking is a way of relaxing."

I know other hostesses who are more into presentation than preparation, but that does not preclude a delicious meal.

Marie-Louise de Clermont-Tonnerre, *Directrice de Societe* for Chanel, and a Frenchwoman of a certain age, is one of the first people I met when I arrived in France all those years ago. She is, as one would imagine, elegant and interesting. She has a magnificent apartment overlooking the Palais Royal gardens where she likes to do dinners for eight. She finds setting a beautiful table to be relaxing.

However, her predilection tends to be more for searching out the best of the best for her parties than preparing a meal herself.

"I'm surrounded by purveyors of extraordinary products," she says. "Receiving is easy in France because it's always possible to find wonderful food and excellent wine. I keep my dinners uncomplicated and always set a pretty table," she adds.

Instead of going to her local pâtisserie for a delectable dessert, on occasion Marie-Louise may turn to one of our—meaning every Frenchwoman and woman I know and *moi-même*—favorite emporiums, Picard, the truly unbelievable frozen-food store chain that has everything anyone could ever imagine (and more) to produce a remarkable meal. From hors d'oeuvres and seafood to sauces that make it seem as if one is an accomplished cook to good breads and marvelous desserts, let's just say it's an amazing place. I am willing to wager that there is not one Frenchwoman in this country who hasn't turned to Picard for an assist in her kitchen.

My interior designer friend Jeanne-Aelia Desparmet-Hart, world traveler and wonderful hostess, says she loves to keep entertaining simple (you see, it's a theme) so that she can spend the maximum amount of time with her guests. I asked her to tell me some of her favorite ways to entertain, and since I found what she said not only interesting, but also worth emulating, I thought I would share with you.

Like Anne-Françoise, Jeanne-Aelia has her first course on the table when guests sit down, which makes for the smooth continuation of the evening from cocktails to dinner.

"For formal entertaining, depending upon the season, I'll serve oysters on a bed of white beans or pretty pink Himalayan salt—for stability—or a slice of foie gras on toasted *pain d'épiceé* (gingerbread) with caramelized onions on top.

"I keep cooking to a minimum," she says.

"The main dish can be osso buco or *blanquette de veau*. I always serve dishes that can be cooked ahead of time for two reasons: cooking odors and time out of the kitchen. I always serve salad and cheese.

"Dessert can be *mousse au chocolat* or poached pears with star-anise syrup. Again, something easily made ahead of time. And then I go all-out for the decor!"

Whether entertaining formally or informally Jeanne-Aelia always assembles inventive, uncomplicated menus.

"In the summer, I serve gazpacho with crushed watermelon in it, with sides of diced cucumber and tomato and small croutons, or some kind of fresh vegetable soup like cucumber with a tiny bit of crushed pineapple or mint," she says.

"I often choose mozzarella—always *bufala*—with sliced tomatoes and a tiny bit of black-olive tapenade.

"An all-season choice can be simplified eggs Benedict: artichoke hearts with smoked salmon and Hollandaise sauce. In winter, I'll opt for hot soups like cauliflower with a tiny bit of cream or individual quiches. For the main course, I'll go again for a ready-to-serve dish like couscous when I feel a bit more exotic, or chicken with dried apricots.

"Dessert might be *crème de marron* with crème fraîche or cream cheese with a coulis of raspberries or plum jam, or some great sorbet, for example.

"I often refer to Marmiton.com for recipes, but for *blanquette de veau,* I have religiously counted on *The Joy of Cooking.* It's perfection.

"I have made a few mistakes and had a few catastrophes, like going too far with the exotic spices or overcooking a dish, but all in all, as long as I can make the meal a good reason to be with friends and family and be creative in the dish and the decor, I am happy."

THE WINE

If in doubt about wine, consulting with an expert at a good wine shop solves the problem. I rely on my husband. I also love talking to sommeliers in restaurants about their favorite wines and how they like to combine them with various foods. I've never met one who wasn't pleased to offer advice.

As one might imagine, David Biraud, the chief sommelier at the five-star Mandarin Oriental Hotel in Paris and vice-champion of the world of *Sommellerie*, is passionate about his métier, but he is not a chauvinist and seeks out new experiences with wines from other countries. "I like to travel around the world for tastings," he says. "I enjoy sampling wines grown and produced in different ways with different climates and growing conditions—it's fascinating for me."

As a journalist, I always hope I'll learn something new or discover something totally unexpected, and in my interview with Monsieur Biraud, I most definitely did. He agreed with Éric Fréchon that many cheeses should be eaten with white wines. "About 99 percent of cheeses should be paired with a white wine," he says. "It's a shame, for example, to drink fine, old reds with a Camembert or Brie."

One of my favorite interviews was with the adorable Jean-André Charial, owner of the luxurious Baumanière hotel and the restaurant's two-star Michelin chef in Provence. He and his talented wife, Geneviève, spoil guests throughout the spring, summer, and early fall before moving to the glorious Le Strato boutique hotel nestled in the Alps in the painfully chic Courchevel ski station.

In one of our conversations, I asked him to tell me a couple of his favorite cheese-and-wine couplings. He says he likes a Sancerre *blanc* with chèvre; a Bordeaux with Saint-Nectaire, specifically Château Haut-Bailly, a Graves; and a Sauternes with Roquefort.

THE MAGIC OF AMBIENCE

Not long ago, Françoise Dumas invited me to a dinner she had arranged in the Musée d'Orsay on a Monday night when the museum was closed to the public. The evening was a "friends of the museum" benefit, and our hostess was the stunning Jacqueline de Ribes.

No cheese as you can see. Since the dinner was on a Monday, it was assumed that many of the invitees worked the next day and wouldn't wish to stay for hours at table.

On the
MENU

ENTRÉE (APPETIZER)
White asparagus with a
creamy sauce

PLAT (MAIN COURSE)
Mignon of veal with spring
vegetables

DESSERT
Two types of strawberries
with basil foam

WINES:
2016 Mouton Cadet Blanc and
2004 Château d'Armailhac

"Shorter dinner parties have been the trend over the last few years," Françoise says. "On a weeknight, almost everyone wants to be home by eleven p.m."

The event began with a tour of the Paul Cézanne exhibit, followed by Champagne on the roof of the museum, and dinner in a gilded private salon. As we entered the large room, we saw a swath of round tables covered in russet cloths, plates rimmed in gold, three etched crystal glasses, white napkins, and, in the center of each table, a large, low bouquet of lush tone-on-tone coral peonies and roses and leaves all seemingly transported directly from a country garden and plunked haphazardly into round, burnished gold vases. Scattered around the base of the vases were clusters of votive candles nestled among small apples of various colors and bunches of green grapes to echo Cézanne's still-life paintings.

You see: entertaining from the simple to the sublime, but always realized with care and attention. Some of my more inventive table settings have been inspired by modified versions of what I've seen at sumptuous dinner parties decorated by famed interior designers collaborating with the most masterful florists in Paris.

Jeanne-Aelia says that when she entertains more formally, she simply amps up the decoration.

"My version of formal is more silverware, more fancy glasses, and embroidered linens. I also splurge on a lot of flowers, and I bring out the larger candlesticks," she says.

"Formal table settings are often white tablecloths and napkins, crystal glasses, good silver, and relatively unadorned plates—though I like to use fun appetizer plates and equally unique dessert plates or bowls. I have never had, nor wished to have, a full set of dishes. It's like wearing one designer head to toe or matching bedroom furniture; it's boring to me.

"I usually start by looking at what I own and get my inspiration from that. I always need a theme. For a red table, I might start with my Murano glasses that have orangey-red stripes and then, for example, choose plates with a large raspberry-red border and a different shade of red linen napkins. Next come linen place mats, sometimes white, sometimes pale blue. To echo the tone-on-tone reds, I use pieces of red coral as knife holders. Then I usually put yellow flowers or plain greenery at the center of the table. If I don't place a bright yellow double candlestick, I'll construct a grouping of five or six Danish white porcelain–and–gold metal candleholders that look quite modern.

"However I set the table, I like it to be eclectic, mixing styles and eras high and low. I serve soup in ice cream bowls with stems and dessert on small plates placed on large exotic leaves if it fits the look. (I have a very creative flower shop near me.) Some of my friends are very innovative in their table settings, using hand-painted plates, colored glasses from here and there, and antique salt-and-pepper shakers in ivory and ebony."

INSPIRATION IS EVERYWHERE and, again, we can be creative no matter our means.

We are lucky to have a large garden where I can always find something to add to a last-minute table setting, regardless of the season. In early spring, there are forsythia and lilacs—both white and mauve—then come the rhododendrons, hydrangeas, roses, peonies, honeysuckles, and lavender. Moving into late fall and winter, the Red Robin bushes have their shiny red-and-green leaves and small clusters of tiny white flowers; other bushes produce lovely red berries; and from our pine trees come literally hundreds of pine cones. At the far end of our garden, I scoop up the masses of Queen Anne's lace in the summer and add the delicate weeds to give a charming airiness to bouquets.

We have ancient pine trees in the garden, which give me a bountiful supply of boughs for Noël, and many of our trees have mistletoe, which I didn't realize was a parasite until a friend told me. Still, it makes for pretty arrangements.

In the fields behind our house, I find stalks of wheat and poppies. In the Rambouillet Forest that surrounds our village, there are masses of wildflowers and all sorts of branches on the ground that we're allowed to collect. I'll use some in arrangements, though not necessarily on the dining table itself because the branches are so much more dramatic when they are in high groupings that would make for difficult conversations across the table. One Noël, I cleaned and sprayed the branches silver and white and let them fall into place in a large unpolished silver-plated urn. The effect was festive and dramatic, so I kept them on display until March.

As I've mentioned, I don't like artificial flowers, nor do my friends. However, Catherine Muller, the brilliant Parisian floral designer and teacher, showed me how fetching branches with and without berries mixed with

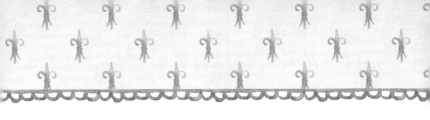

Wine: Enhancing the EXPERIENCE

Drinking wine is a special and complex experience. It's a combination of many things including the right wine, at the right moment, in the right place, with the right person. There is *always* an element of ambience in the pleasure derived from wine.

In order to understand the nuances that enhance the pleasure of wine consumption, I asked David Biraud to share some of his tips and secrets.

- Pouilly-Fuissé is one of my favorite wines, and he told me it is excellent with meat. Often the French will refuse to drink a white wine with meat—I live with one such Frenchman. In fact, he drinks red wine with everything, from fish to cheese, and has no intention of exploring the myriad possibilities of white wine.

- "Madeira, sherry, and Champagne are always excellent aperitif choices," Biraud says. My unasked question was, When is Champagne *ever* not an excellent choice?

- Biraud began building his *cave* as a young man, carefully studying the qualities of each year's regions and their potential for becoming great wines in the future. "When building one's own *cave,* be patient," he says. It often takes time for wines to mature into their potential for greatness."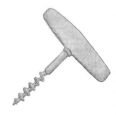

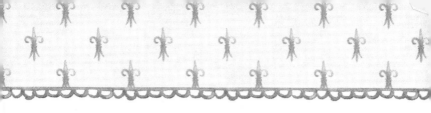

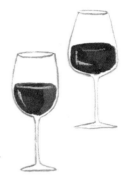

- The very act of collecting wines is a great adventure, he tells me. The personality and tastes of a collector figure into the choices, which add another layer of pleasure. Each wine can have a story: how you found it, why you like it, how you serve it.

- Many of us think of rosés as solely summer wines, but according to Biraud, we are missing out on the delicious pairing of rosés with game birds.

- "Rieslings," he notes, "pair nicely with smoked mackerel."

- True wine aficionados agree that an element of utmost importance when drinking wine is that one must be able to see and appreciate its color. Therefore, they say, wineglasses should be transparent. In fact, Biraud says all the better if the glasses are of the finest crystal, "because it gives the best wine-drinking experience."

- For those of us who like the idea of using colorful wineglasses for their undeniable decorative effect, Biraud feels we should reject the impulse (though we still have the option of choosing a gold, silver, or colored rim or a colorful stem).Happily, Biraud loves Champagne and has a particular affinity for rosé Champagnes. "They have more texture," he says, "and they're friendly and festive. No one can cry when drinking pink Champagne."

long stems of silk forsythia or apple blossoms could change my mind. She did indeed, but not for faux floral bouquets or faux plants, which she doesn't like either.

The rest of the branch harvest we use for kindling along with pine cones.

Nothing says cozy entertaining like a crackling fire in the fireplace. In late fall and winter, we always begin a dinner party with Champagne in front of the fire and finish the evening there with coffee, tisanes, and chocolates. When it's just the two of us, my husband and I will often have dinner in the living room in front of the fire on cold, dreary nights.

For a New Year's Eve party one year, Anne-Françoise placed small, round silver-plated picture frames with our names written in silver ink inside to mark our places. At the end of the evening, she gave them to us as New Year's presents.

Christine Guérard is a romantic at heart and sets her tables accordingly. "As a child, I loved fairy tales, and I've tried never to lose that sense of wonder and imagination in those stories," she says. On the table I was seated at, she had placed a burnished-bronze rabbit, a tiny antique wooden birdcage with its door open, a terra-cotta pot of roses, votive candles, and small yellow and red apples here and there, all on a round table covered in a floor-skimming skirt of beige linen and a tablecloth in variegated beige-and-white stripes.

"I think if we're not romantic, it's not possible to do anything extraordinary," she says. "We have to dream."

THE ELEMENTS OF THE TABLE

As you have no doubt ascertained at this point, I am fascinated by *l'art de table*. My interest revolves around its origins and protocols—a few once-acceptable behaviors are quite surprising, even shocking for us today—and how conventions have evolved over the centuries.

From my observations and extensive research, I've learned that apart from the gradual refinement of etiquette *à table* (no host or hostess places one goblet to be shared by everyone around a dining table, for example), the history, usages, and rituals of dining are an intriguing way to understand the traditions and aesthetic predilections of a culture.

Since I had so much fun on my historical quest, I thought you too might enjoy my discoveries. Beginning with the concept of a specific room for dining and continuing to the glasses, flatware, plates, linens, etiquette, and more, here are some of my favorite findings:

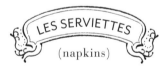

LES SERVIETTES
(napkins)

As with everything associated with *l'art de recevoir à la française,* a fascinating history precedes its modern incarnation. Without tracing its origins all the way back to the Roman Empire, I'll start with its evolution in France. During the Middle Ages, the edge of the tablecloth that spilled over the side onto the diners' laps when seated at table was used to wipe the mouth and hands. Later a large, sheet-size cloth was hung in a corner of the room where diners were eating. When they felt the need, they used the communal cloth to wipe their hands and mouth.

During the Renaissance, linen napkins lightly perfumed with rosewater became part of elegant households. They were huge compared to even the largest napkins we have today.

In the nineteenth century, decoration was added to the fabric in the form of embroidery and lace, which signaled a certain social status. By the beginning of the twentieth century, beautiful napkins, often hand-embroidered, along with tablecloths became part of a young woman's trousseau—the continuation of a family's patrimony meant to be passed on to future generations.

Some hostesses maintain that napkins can be placed either on the table or on the plates for lunches, but for a more formal dinner, they should not obscure the plates, which may be more precious or elaborately decorated. Therefore, the idea is that napkins should be on the table to the left of the forks. Françoise Dumas, however, has taken the lead from her mentor, the Countess de Ribes, and always puts napkins on the plates.

"When the napkin comes off the plate, it's a lovely discovery to see what's beneath," she says. When the hostess is seated and takes her napkin, that is the signal that the guests follow her lead.

A napkin is never completely unfolded when placed on the lap, and never, ever, I'm told, should a napkin be placed in a glass.

La Salle à Manger
THE DINING ROOM

The dining room, as in a room specifically designed for the consumption of meals, is a relatively new concept—new by historical measure, that is.

In the Middle Ages, the expression *dresser la table* meant to "set up the table" as opposed to "set the table." Dining tables were "set up," as in moved from place to place depending upon the seasons and perhaps the whims of a dwelling's inhabitants. The maneuver involved placing a large plank of wood on wooden supports, attractively camouflaged with fabric reaching to the floor and decorated in accordance with the wealth and station of the family.

The seventeenth century saw the beginning of dining rooms becoming part of new château construction, but it wasn't until the eighteenth century that the trend began to capture the imagination of a larger public.

When you think about it, there is something romantic and refreshing about moving dining locations in the house and around the garden. Placing a table in front of a fireplace in winter is charming, dining in a book-lined library is elegant, and a table for two *en amoureux* in a bedroom is another idea from the past. Why not?

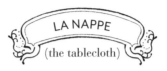

LA NAPPE
(the tablecloth)

A protective pad always goes beneath tablecloths, not only to safeguard against spills and hot serving pieces, but also because it adds a certain comfort, softens the look of the cloth, and adds another elegant detail to the table.

At minimum, the tablecloth should descend twelve inches all around and can fall close to the seat of the chair or to the floor for the utmost elegance. When the tablecloth falls to the floor, the chairs should be pulled back slightly from the table so as not to "break" the fall of the material. Placing another cloth over the floor-skimming one adds another layer of chic to the ensemble.

Boutis, lightweight bed coverings made with a lovely Provençal quilting technique that results in a *matelassé* finish, make lovely table coverings. They have a rustic-chic allure that can be dressed up or down.

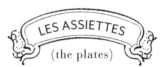

LES ASSIETTES
(the plates)

So much of the refinement of *l'art de table* began with noble families, and over the centuries it became more democratic and available to all of us.

The first plates in pewter, silver, and gold were on the tables of wealthy families, while poor families ate from pottery bowls until as late as the turn of the twentieth century in some regions. By the eighteenth century, however, faience plates—in varying degrees of sophistication—were widely accessible.

For the ultimate comfort around a table, plates should be placed slightly less than one inch from the edge of the table and between twelve to sixteen inches between each person (all of this assumes the table will accommodate the measures).

The *assiette de presentation*, or charger, always adds a further refined detail to the table. It can be simple in rattan or elaborate in silver, part of a set of china, or something completely whimsical in painted glass or papier-mâché.

Doris Brynner loves painted-glass plates and had charming designs made for the Dior Maison collections.

We always have an entrée with our meals, whether or not we're entertaining. A normal, everyday dinner for the two of us includes three plates: an entrée, a main course, and a dessert.

When we're entertaining, each place has the charger, the dinner plate, and on top of it the small plate for the first course, the entrée. I don't use chargers for the two of us unless we're celebrating something. The charger is removed after the main course and before the cheese if one chooses to serve *fromage*. We might have cheese once a week as a special treat.

As for a bread dish, to the left above the forks, I occasionally include them in my entertaining. They're useful and attractive. Note that if one is not provided, the

French place their bread, once taken from the serving tray, to the left on the table, not on the dinner plate.

We usually serve cheese at dinner parties, which requires another plate and then a dessert plate or bowl and plate. If I don't place the appropriate knives, forks, and spoons for those courses on the table above the plates before the party, I'll arrange each grouping on a sideboard in the dining room.

Ice creams and sorbets are eaten with forks in France, and a spoon is used to scoop up what may have melted in the bottom of the bowl. What can I say?

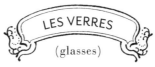

Coffee cups and teacups with their saucers, small spoons, and a sugar bowl wait on a tray in the kitchen to be transported into the living room. No French person I know puts milk in coffee after breakfast, but since I do, I put a small pitcher of milk on the tray.

Coffee and tisanes are not served at the dining table unless, as Albane de Maigret, etiquette expert and professor of *les bonnes manières*, points out, "everyone is participating in a riveting conversation and you, the hostess, don't want to interrupt the ambience. Then maybe you'll quickly ask if your guests would like coffee at the table without breaking the rhythm of the exchange."

LES VERRES
(glasses)

In the seventeenth century, one glass was shared by everyone at the table. In wealthier households, three or four glasses were shared. In the late eighteenth century, manufacturers began to produce glasses of different sizes for specific uses, but it wasn't until the nineteenth century that an assortment of glasses began to be routinely placed on dining tables in what the French call service *à la russe*. The difference between service *à la russe* versus service *à la française* is that in the first instance each course is served sequentially, which means food is plated in the kitchen, whereas usually in France serving pieces are on the table and passed, allowing guests to serve themselves. This allows everyone to decide the serving size they prefer. If the evening includes personnel serving at table (from the left), the

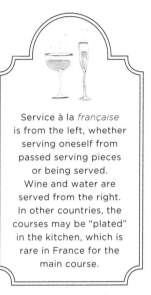

Service à la *française* is from the left, whether serving oneself from passed serving pieces or being served. Wine and water are served from the right. In other countries, the courses may be "plated" in the kitchen, which is rare in France for the main course.

same "self service" applies. Restaurants almost always employ service *à la russe*.

The order of glasses, descending from left to right, is: water in the largest, red wine in a smaller glass, and white wine in a still smaller glass. The Champagne glass is arranged slightly behind and to the right of the water glass.

Water glasses are already filled when everyone arrives at the table.

NOW THE BIG QUESTION IS, should Champagne be served in flutes or in coupes? From an aesthetic point of view, both are lovely, but the experts believe that neither form does justice to its festive effervescence.

"With a flute you can't get all of the perfume, and a coupe is a horror—you lose all the bubbles, and it's the bubbles that make Champagne so exciting and festive," says Carol Duval-Leroy, proprietor of the excellent Duval-Leroy Champagne house. "A tulip-shaped glass is always the best choice for the ultimate Champagne experience."

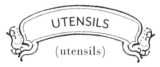

UTENSILS
(utensils)

Everyone knows how to place knives, forks, and spoons on a dining table, and everyone knows that we work from the outside in when using them. However, what everyone may not know is that in France, the fork and spoon are placed facedown because the monograms and the silver stamps are on what many of us consider the back of the utensil.

More and more, we're seeing tables in restaurants, though not in French homes, with the tines of the fork and the bowl of the spoon facing up. Albane de Maigret regrets seeing this tendency, "even in some three-star restaurants," she says. She is a stickler for tradition.

Over the centuries, additional purpose-made eating utensils were added to the repertoire of refined tables. Fish knives and forks, for instance, entered the panoply in the nineteenth century.

The knife, fork, and spoon for cheese and dessert may be placed above the plates on the table. I remember the direction in which they are to be arranged because they point in the opposite direction. Starting from the top, the cheese-knife blade points toward the forks on the left of the plate; beneath the cheese knife is the dessert spoon, bowl facing the forks, and finally the dessert fork, tines directed toward the knives. In France, the tines and bowl of the spoon face the table. *Et voilà!*

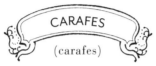

CARAFES

(carafes)

In France, the hostess, as the "*chef d'orchestre*," as Françoise Dumas says, has plenty to do, so happily everything that revolves around wine and water is the host's job or can be assigned to one of the male guests if there isn't a male host in the house.

Depending upon the wine, the amount of time it should be opened before serving varies. At minimum, a red wine should be opened twenty minutes before serving and a white ten minutes, so they can breathe. Again, turn to an expert if in doubt. The bottle, unless you're serving an old and perhaps precious wine that might need decanting, should be placed on the table in an attractive holder so that everyone can see the label. Furthermore, the holder will prevent errant drops from staining the table or the tablecloth.

Men serve the wine in France. It is their job to watch guests to make certain no one sits before an empty glass. (One never puts a hand over a glass to refuse a serving or a refill.)

The host first pours a small amount of wine in his glass to taste before serving others to assure the wine is not corked.

If there are no men, all my friends agree that wine is served by the person closest to the bottle or carafe.

I recently discovered that pouring wine into a carafe—which is not the same as decanting—is for young wines, whether white or red. If for aesthetic reasons or for aeration you like the idea of pretty carafes, the empty bottles should be placed on a buffet or side table where guests can see what they are drinking. Most likely the host will explain, but in France everyone likes to read wine labels.

As for water, it is always more appealing to have one or more carafes on the table. There is nothing pretty about water bottles. Mineral waters, whether fizzy or flat, can be served from carafes, usually by the host (or surrogate host), who refills glasses when he sees someone needs more water.

We're allowed to ask for more water, but we have to be patient if we desire more wine. Albane de Maigret says that there has been a "loosening" of the rules for water. It's not the end of the world if a woman pours water.

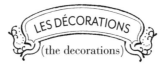

LES DÉCORATIONS
(the decorations)

Flowers, flowers, flowers, of course, but not those loved for their beautiful perfumes on a dining table. Avoid jasmine, particularly fragrant roses, freesia, some camellias, and lilies. Stéphane Bern, France's beloved expert on all things royal and refined, tells me he was invited to a dinner where the table was festooned with mimosas.

"The minute we sat down, we were engulfed in the fragrance, and I *knew* the dinner wasn't going to be good," he says.

"Was it?" I ask him. "No, it wasn't," he says, laughing.

Whether in the form of candelabra, candlesticks, hurricane lamps, or votive candles, there is nothing quite so flattering, romantic, and lovely as the subtle glow from candlelight. The flames should be above eye level to obtain the maximum benefits from the reflection. The flames should never be low to the table, excluding votives, of course, because they cast an unflattering upward shadow that is not complimentary to even the youngest guests.

On the subject of candles, the second a candle goes into a holder—or any place in the house, for that matter—the wick must be "tipped." That means all wicks on display should be black, no naked wicks. It also makes for easier lighting of the candles when setting the table.

As for other tabletop ideas, be as simple or extravagant as your mood dictates. Many years ago, a Parisian friend scattered iridescent white and gray "pearls" down the middle of her table interspersed with votive candles in mercury-glass holders, three multibranched silver candelabra, and mercury-glass vases filled with white and pale pink peonies. Her tablecloth and napkins were a light pearl gray; her plates white, rimmed in silver; water goblets were silver; and the delicate wineglasses clear and again rimmed in silver. Her table was breathtaking.

I've discovered marvelous arts-and-crafts stores in Paris and Versailles that are full of potential table decorations. My friend found her "pearls" in a tiny shop in Paris when she was looking for an indoor winter project for her granddaughter.

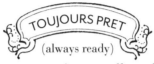

No matter how we entertain, casually or formally or a bit of both, it's best to be prepared. When our table coverings, napkins, candles, decorations, plates, and glasses are arranged logically and set up for easy access, half of the challenge of entertaining is solved.

Terry de Gunzburg, the chic and talented creator of the luxury cosmetic collection By Terry, opened her many glass, china, and silver closets for me to demonstrate how she has arranged each collection in the ways she likes to mix and match the elements for her parties. The instant you look at the shelves, ideas pop into your head of how certain plates would look with others and how the crystal would add a sparkling dimension. Then she has a collection of small "suitcases" filled with Yves Saint Laurent's silver, stored just below. Linens are carefully arranged in another area.

Anne-Françoise is, as I've mentioned, probably the most well-organized person I have ever known. Her armoires, linen closets, crystal cabinets, china closets, silver cases, and decorative objects all have their assigned places, and everything always returns where it belongs.

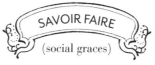

SAVOIR FAIRE
(social graces)

We all learned our etiquette at the table as children and have done our best to pass along the finer points of civilized dining to our children and grandchildren, exactly the way French families do.

When I was a child my mother, who was not the world's best cook, always set a lovely dinner table that included candles and flowers. It was in that setting that my father, with whom I had a reciprocal adoration, insisted that I learn good table manners.

In France, there are a few more imperatives at the table that I've observed over the years, for example, the way to cut cheese properly and to not cut salad. Let me share a few discoveries with you.

- The time generally allotted to cocktails is about forty-five minutes.
- In France we "dine" or "have lunch," *diner* or *déjeuner*, while *manger*, "to eat," is used when followed by what one consumes. I ate an apple; I ate a piece of cake, etc.
- No touching glasses in toasts, just a raised glass and a meaningful gaze. The clinking of glasses began in the Middle Ages when goblets were heartily slammed against each other. The idea was that if

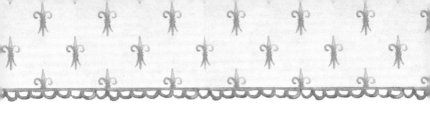

Comment Manger Le Fromage
HOW TO EAT CHEESE

To assure the ultimate pleasure from each type, I turned to our *fromager*, Monsieur LeBris, for advice. This is what he told me:

- **IF SERVING A CHEESE COURSE:** The platter can feature one perfect offering like a Brie de Meaux, but if you wish to give guests choices, the minimum number is three (it should always be an odd number). Depending upon one's source of reference, there are between 350 and 400 types of cheese in France.

- **LET IT REST:** Cover the platter with a moist tea towel and let the cheeses "rest" for approximately one hour before they are served. Make certain the cheeses are separated so there is no transfer of taste. To release its subtle (or not so subtle) flavors, like wine, cheese needs to breathe.

- **THE HEART:** Ideally, each cheese should have its own knife. When cutting from a wedge of cheese, like Brie or Roquefort, slice from the back to the point. The point, which is the "heart" of the cheese, is considered the best part and is not to be lopped off so others cannot enjoy it.

- **CORRECT ORDER:** The cheeses are best consumed from the mild to the strong so that our palate can appreciate the personality of each *fromage*.

- **SERVE ONCE:** Unless you are among close friends and family, you may only serve yourself once—no second helpings. It is also considered rude to try all of the cheeses.

- **EVER SO GENTLY:** Even soft cheeses are to be placed on bread, not spread like butter. A quick "press down" with our cheese knife should ensure it stays on the bread.

> *"How do you expect anyone to govern a country that has more than 258 varieties of cheese?"*
> —Charles de Gaulle

A CHEESE PLATE LINE-UP TO CONSIDER:

1. Chèvre and Brebis (goat and sheep cheese)
2. Brie, Camembert, Coulommiers
3. Cantal, Mimolette, Tomme de Savoie, Reblochon
4. Beaufort, Emmental, Comté
5. Pont l'Evêque, Munster
6. Roquefort, Bleu d'Auvergne

AND THIS ONE FROM MY NEW FRIEND, CHEF JEAN-ANDRÉ CHARIAL:

1. Chèvre *frais* (a soft, fresh goat cheese that is very mild)
2. Brie
3. St. Nectaire
4. Chèvre *sec* (a dry goat cheese that becomes harder and stronger with age)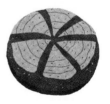
5. Roquefort, Fourme d'Ambert

there were poison in one of the vessels, it would spill over into the other goblet, a sort of test to see if your friend wanted to kill you. At least that was more civilized than having a resident poison tester.

~ Salad is to be "folded" with the help of a small morsel of bread, which is rather tricky, but most thoughtful hostesses make certain lettuce is broken into bite-size pieces. If the fold method isn't working, cut with the edge of a fork.

~ It's time to banish these two words from our vocabulary: *Bon appétit*. The salutation that translates literally as "good appetite" actually refers to the good function of the digestive system, as in the intestines. Not particularly appetizing, *n'est-ce pas*?

~ Bread is broken by hand into small, bite-size pieces and is used only to "assist" food onto a fork, *never* to sop up a sauce on a plate.

~ When the meal is finished and the hostess suggests everyone move to the salon for coffee and tisanes, napkins are placed to the left of the plate, unfolded, exactly the way Americans do it.

~ Coffee and tea are not served with dessert. They are the final course of the meal and rarely served at the table.

There are other nuances to the French dinner party. "*L'exactitude est la politesse des rois*," ("Punctuality is the courtesy of kings"), was the only gift a king could give his subjects as a mark of respect, but when it comes to guests arriving to a dinner at the precise hour of the invitation, that's simply not done. Guests are supposed to give their hosts and hostesses a fifteen-minute grace period. An invitation for 8 p.m. means 8:15ish.

An American friend of mine who has lived in France more than forty years told me that when she first moved here, she and her husband arrived at a black-tie dinner in a Parisian hotel at precisely eight. "We spent thirty minutes drinking Champagne with the waitstaff before the French started to arrive," she says. "Live and learn."

As far as how to greet your fellow guests, for the ubiquitous air-kiss greeting, keep it to two (one for each cheek). Unless one is familiar with the technique involved in *le baisemain*, the kiss on the hand that Frenchmen sometimes perform, it's probably best left to the experts. It's not as easy as it looks, and it involves a list of dos and don'ts, one of which is that the lips *effleurer,* or lightly brush the hand. In other words, it's not really a kiss. And one is not *enchanté*, or enchanted, to meet someone. We may be pleased or delighted or happy, but *enchanted* means a spell has been cast upon us, and furthermore it's an adjective. If you look up the word, you'll see that it has morphed into a new meaning, but purists vociferously object. (OK, one could quibble, but that's the way it is.)

Should you bring a gift? According to Albane de Maigret, arriving to dinners with a gift is a relatively new trend. "It's not at all necessary—or expected—to arrive with a gift. The idea is that one is happy with the presence of guests, and a *cadeau* is not part of the ritual," she says. At a later date, the invitees most likely will extend a reciprocal invitation to their hosts. However, invitees can send flowers to their hostess the day before her party or the day after. As we know, one never arrives with flowers in hand. And it's not unusual to see guests arrive with a small box of excellent chocolates, a discreet offering that is then shared among the group with coffee.

After a special evening, it's charming to write a *lettre de château*, a thank-you note. For simple get-togethers, a day-after text message or telephone call is always appreciated.

THE GUESTS

The right mélange of guests is the essential element that contributes to the special alchemy that one always hopes will envelop the atmosphere.

That, too, requires a certain finesse, and no one knows that better than Françoise Dumas, who has spent decades arranging the seating at party tables. She can spend days thinking about whom to seat next to whom for an enjoyable evening, and conversely how to separate guests who have unresolved issues.

At one party, she placed me between a former American ambassador to France and a world-famous wine critic. I had the most fantastic time. (I should mention that generous servings of exceptional wine were involved, since the soiree was held under a huge tent in the vineyards of Château Mouton Rothschild in Bordeaux.)

At the end of the evening, I thanked Françoise profusely for the kindness and thoughtfulness that went into my place at table. "I thought you would enjoy yourself, and I'm so glad you did," she said.

As the executive director of the French-American Chamber of Commerce in Chicago, my daughter is responsible for arranging two large annual benefits. She told me that after she and her staff spent a week making the seating plan for a black-tie dinner, she was shocked to see people moving the strategically arranged place cards so they could sit next to spouses or friends. In France, couples are separated at the table, and it would be more than surprising to see someone changing the seating arrangements.

Naturally, most of us are not involved in precision-placement conundrums—I'm certainly not—but introducing new friends to longtime friends is a wonderful way to entertain, and mixing up the group so that everyone can discover something interesting in the context of animated conversation can result in unforgettable encounters.

A few years ago, we invited English friends for dinner who had expressed interest in meeting another friend of ours whose brother was in the French Resistance during World War II. We had him and his wife, a journalist, for an extraordinary evening that lasted well into the early morning.

Exchanging ideas, sharing points of view, learning something surprising, and meeting someone with whom one discovers a natural affinity can be the serendipitous result of a shared meal.

So how many guests to invite? Almost everyone I interviewed liked the magic number eight.

Le Role des Meilleures Hostesses:
THE ROLE OF THE BEST HOSTESSES

Here are a few tips from Françoise Dumas who assembles some of the most spectacularly unforgettable parties in France, Monaco, and beyond:

- Who doesn't love that "wow" moment when you walk into a dining room? It's not at all difficult, but it means everything to your guests. Go for harmony, a theme; entertaining does not have to be elaborate or complicated.

- Even for simple dinners for six, eight, or ten, have a seating plan memorized or on a Post-it for your own review before everyone arrives. Place cards can help dispel any confusion.

- We all know the boy-girl-boy-girl setup is best when possible.

- Place a quiet, introverted guest next to a talker who will ask questions and start a conversation. In general, separate talkers and non-talkers.

- When mixing old friends with new, separate the old friends so they don't fall into familiar conver-sations that could exclude others.

- Try to place guests who share similar affinities, like travel or antiques or dogs or fine wine, next to one another.

- And on the contrary, separate people you know have strong opposingopinions that could erupt during a conversation and make the evening unpleasant for all. In France, taboo subjects include religion, money, and politics. When the group is in general agreement about politics, though, the topic may be discussed—sometimes at length.

- Separate couples, but not fiancés or newlyweds of a year or less. (Isn't that sweet?)

- Never change the place "assigned" by the hostess unless you ask her permission. She had her reasons for arranging her table, and she probably took considerable time deciding how she could use the seating to enhance the ambience of the evening.

- Round tables tend to be the most convivial because they don't relegate guests to faraway places where it can be difficult to hear and participate in conversations.

Le Rôle des Bons Invités:
THE ROLE OF GOOD GUESTS

Entertaining is not a one-sided affair. Guests, too, have their part to play, otherwise all the good intentions and efforts of the hostess are in vain. Surely when receiving, we choose our guests with their attributes in mind so that everyone shares a *bon moment.* **Some worthwhile tips:**

- A good guest is happy to be included.

- Sit properly at the table—do not slouch or rest on your elbows.

- "Dress for the occasion, be well-mannered, watch your posture, and come in a good mood," says Mathilde Favier. "I want to be surrounded by smart, happy people. It's the only way to have fun."

- If someone has nothing to say, we forget he or she Is present. When you are a guest, it is important to come prepared to contribute to conversations.

- Speak to the person on your right and on your left. A good guest never favors one over the other, says Albane de Maigret. "And remember, a conversation is not a monologue. Fifty percent of an exchange is listening."

- Doris Brynner's advice is, "If you don't know what to say, ask questions."

- Do not even think about putting a telephone on the table. A good guest never takes pictures at the table and posts nothing to social media during the meal (nor after, without explicit permission).

- Flirting is perfectly acceptable when, as Stéphane Bern says, "no red lines are crossed."

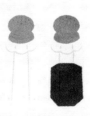

Over the years I've become not only comfortable, but also happy, in the role of hostess, although I have never had a sit-down dinner party for more than eight. My husband prefers six because he thinks the conversation is better. "With eight," he maintains, "there tends to be two conversations; with six, normally everyone participates in one conversation." I actually prefer more than one conversation around a dinner table for at least part of an evening. It signals that guests are sharing stories and experiences and, I hope, having fun.

"I love to do a dinner party for eight with just the right mix of people on Thursday evenings because it's almost the weekend and there is something celebratory about a Thursday," Mathilde Favier says. "I invite people to whom I want to listen and from whom I can learn something. It's so rewarding for me to think after an evening that I've learned something new. Don't you agree?"

Yes, I do agree.

"Oh, yes, music is very important," she adds.

Françoise Dumas says the role of the best hostesses, of whom she knows many should be to act like *les chefs d'orchestre*, making sure all elements of a social gathering are in perfect harmony, from the food to the conversation. "It's a job, in a way—a good hostess watches everything. Her desire is to make her guests happy for a few hours," she says.

The Perfect
GUEST LIST

Everyone I interviewed had very specific criteria for that prominent supporting-actor role, and the mix of costars who would potentially contribute to a successful occasion. Here is one of Francoise Dumas's hypothetical grand soiree tables:

- AN AMBASSADOR
- AN ACADEMICIAN
- A WRITER
- A BUSINESSMAN OR A BUSINESSWOMAN
- AN ARTIST
- AN INTELLECTUAL
- SOMEONE YOU KNOW WELL FOR THE COMFORT OF FRIENDSHIP
- SOMEONE YOU DO NOT KNOW WELL FOR A NEW DISCOVERY
- SOMEONE BUBBLY TO ADD EFFERVESCENCE TO A TABLE
- A PHILOSOPHER
- A DECORATOR
- A POLITICIAN

Autre Choses
OTHER THINGS

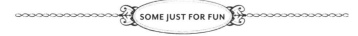

SOME JUST FOR FUN

Since sparkling conversation is the final element that makes an occasion with good food, fine wine, and interesting guests unforgettable, I thought it would be fun to pass along a few French superstitions that could spark a conversation *chez vous*.

❧ Having thirteen at the table is bad luck. In the corner of my friend Anne-Françoise's dining room sits *Monsieur Quatorze* (Mr. Fourteen), made of iron and well-dressed for a party, including a bright yellow waistcoat. She adds him whenever she ends up wth thirteen for dinner. The superstition comes from the Bible, when Judas betrayed Christ.

❧ Bread must never be placed upside down on a table, because this was the way bread was given from the *boulangers* to executioners during the *Ancien Régime.*

❧ When passing the salt, it is never given hand to hand, but rather slid—some say "pushed"—next to the person who requested it.

❧ When moving into a new home, take the dining table in first to ensure good fortune in your new abode.

❧ If a chair is knocked over when leaving the table, that means someone told a lie during the meal.

❧ If you break a crystal glass, good luck will follow. (Though perhaps not in the opinion of the person who owned the glass.)

❧ If you are served the last drop of wine, you will marry in the year or have a baby. (You can see how this is often apocryphal.)

❧ At midnight, upon the passage of Christmas Eve into Christmas Day, open the doors and windows to let all the bad spirits out of the house.

❧ On New Year's Eve, it's important to empty the last drops in bottles to guarantee good luck in the coming year.

A FEW LAST WORDS

In a recent television documentary on *l'art de vivre à la française,* a reporter asked guests at a large cocktail party in Paris how they would define the concept. With few exceptions, the two words chosen were *elegance* and *conviviality.* Not surprisingly, many went on to qualify and embellish their first responses by adding French cuisine.

What is more convivial than entertaining? Entertaining gives us the opportunity to be creative on myriad levels and then present the results to friends and family. We might be showered with rave reviews.

The more we entertain, the easier and more fun it becomes. Great joy comes from seeing guests truly enjoying themselves in our homes.

If, as so many of us believe, time is our greatest luxury, what better way to spend it than among friends and family around a lovely table with delicious food and superlative conversation?

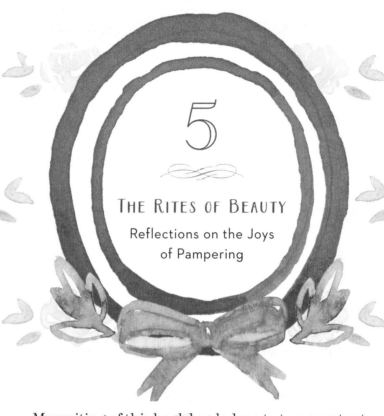

5

THE RITES OF BEAUTY

Reflections on the Joys
of Pampering

My writing of this book has led me to two constant themes within *l'art de vivre à la française:* pleasure and attitude. Together they permeate every aspect of a Frenchwoman's life, from the kitchen to the bedroom to her toilette. (The toilette, as you know, is the pleasant process of dressing and grooming.)

The rites and rituals of beauty routines are an integral part of a Frenchwoman's life. Decades ago, when I began to rethink my approach to skin care and beauty because of what I was seeing with my French girlfriends, I realized and quickly came to appreciate the crucial importance of applying oneself to the process involved in the task.

Frenchwomen enjoy their head-to-toe beauty ministrations, basking in the sensual pleasures of their favorite products while using them, then delighting in the efficacious results. Above all, Frenchwomen, particularly those of a certain age (practice makes perfect), understand that beauty requires investment. Now, for a Frenchwoman that investment usually has little to do with expensive products and everything to do with time. They invest *time* in their beauty routines and, once again, turn their toilette into an enjoyable experience.

Over the centuries, Frenchwomen tending to their beauty rituals have been romantically immortalized in hauntingly beautiful paintings by some of France's most eminent artists. Berthe Morisot, Henri de Toulouse-Lautrec, Pierre Bonnard, and Gustave Caillebotte have, each in their singular styles, captured the very essence of the delicate gestures involved in beauty rituals as the artist's subjects, in a sort of ethereal concentration, were unaware that they were being observed. *L'art de vivre à la française,* indeed.

THE PLEASURE PRINCIPLE

This conscious decision to approach just about everything in life with a positive mind-set is a Frenchwoman's magic formula for happiness. In other words, all it takes is an attitude adjustment to turn effort into enjoyment. Why in the world, they puzzle, when the results of skin care are so obviously positive, wouldn't everyone want to enjoy the time it takes to look better every single day? How can women consider the use of all the wonderful products available to them as tools required for a necessary chore rather than elixirs to enhance an instant of pure indulgence?

Many non-Frenchwomen seem to believe that taking time for themselves is somehow egotistical. But where is the joy in feeling constantly put upon because all we do is take care of others and not ourselves? Ultimately resentment ensues, and we are less happy with our lives. It's important for women to remember that small actions can do wonders for one's mood. It could be as simple as a manicure. When we're happy it shows, and good moods tend to be contagious (as, sadly, do bad moods). As a result, ensuring our own happiness will ensure that of our family as well.

"Put on your lipstick and face the world."

—TERRY DE GUNZBURG

Over the years, I've been asked to describe or define Frenchwomen of a certain age with a few words. These are the adjectives I use:

1) *Pragmatic*

2) *Realistic*

3) *Romantic*

4) *Generous*

5) *Self-possessed* (as in composed)

6) *Self-aware* (very often resulting in self-assurance)

The combination of realism, pragmatism, and romanticism is something I love about my French girlfriends of a certain age and many others that I have interviewed. I think it's their extremely intelligent recipe for a life well lived—they take control and pleasure where they can and accept the ebb and flow of life. *C'est la vie!*

THE SCIENCE OF BEAUTY

All of my friends visit their dermatologists at least once each year for a head-to-toe checkup, or twice if we have specific skin problems. One of my best friends is on a no-soap regime accompanied by rich, fragrance-free creams and lotions to alleviate her serious dry-skin problem.

The Frenchwomen I know educate themselves on the science behind the products they use. I've seen pharmacist Dr. Christine Salort, my great pal, spend considerable time with her clients explaining the benefits of essential oils, no-nonsense products for acne and dry skin, and some of the more "fun" beauty potions on the shelves of her pharmacy. Recently, she gave me a tester for a new La Roche-Posay serum, Hyalu B5, to take home and try (I realize I'm spoiled), then told me I needed the cream that is to be applied after the serum, Hyalu B5 Anti-Wrinkle Care Repairing Replumping. The duo, which has two pure hyaluronic acids and vitamin B5, is to be used day and night.

Here's what I know: I mentioned in my previous book and several times on my blog that Frenchwomen tend to look at their skin-care rituals with a different philosophy than many of us. They expect—no, demand—that the products they use from head to toe are efficacious and want them to fulfill other desires. A gratifying experience, based on myriad criteria, is of primary importance:

- Products must feature serious scientific ingredients with studies that support their alleged results.
- For some, brands that are natural or ecologically friendly, and that offer the basics in exfoliation, cleansing, masks, and moisturizing but eschew chemical components, are more important to a woman's aesthetic.
- Others feel that a lovely fragrance permeating the atmosphere is an essential element of pleasure. I agree when it comes to bath products.

FOR AS LONG AS I CAN REMEMBER, I have loved the marvelous offerings under the broad category of beauty. Maybe it's because the word itself seems like a promise, one in which we can proactively participate.

The definition of that promise has changed significantly during my decades living in France. Now, like many Frenchwomen, I buy all my skin-care and treatment products from the pharmacy, not beauty counters, because they are science based, no-nonsense functional, and highly effective. I have zero interest in pretty packaging around a serum, mask, or moisturizer, and I don't need fragrance in my day or night creams.

Then there is my single prescription skin-care product, which if you have read my previous book, you know is vitamin A cream or Retin-A. I've been using it for almost thirty years and consider it to be a miracle in a tube, as do many dermatologists and even plastic surgeons.

Dr. Valérie Leduc, a generalist by training and a phlebologist (a doctor who specializes in vein disorders, including varicose veins), has converted her broad expertise into a holistic and intimately personal approach to beauty. "In the past, I thought women in their forties were the most beautiful," she says, "but now I think it's women in their fifties and sixties."

Dr. Leduc has a protocol she likes to follow with her patients. She wants to know *everything* about them, including why they think they need her services. "My approach is global, and I spend an hour or more in a complete checkup," she says. "Before treating the exterior, it is essential to understand a patient's fundamental health and quality of life."

When Dr. Leduc has assessed her patients, she can then lead them to a formula for "aging well, good health, and beauty." She has five criteria for a life well lived:

　1) Eat a healthy, varied diet.

　2) Do age-appropriate exercise.

　3)Practice techniques to deal with stress.

　4) Seek out things that make you happy. "Happiness
　　　repairs our DNA, so it's important to discover
　　　how and what makes us happy," she says.

　5) Relaunch your social networks if you have let
　　　them languish. That includes family, friends,
　　　and coworkers.

Now you may be thinking, Of course, we all know those things. Yes we do, but Dr. Leduc's overall approach is different from any other doctor of aesthetic medicine I have read about or met. She doesn't simply *recommend* lifestyle changes, she attempts to assist women in finding the ways and means to accomplish them. On the subject of happiness, she has suggested to patients that they might look into artistic endeavors, like painting or singing.

Many new patients may schedule an appointment with Dr. Leduc simply for a procedure like fillers, dermabrasion, chemical peels, laser treatments, or epilation. Before she does a treatment, she wants to understand her patient's expectations and motivations for desiring the procedure. She hopes she can convince them that together, they can examine a global approach to healthy, happy aging and their overall well-being. She believes that aging well and beauty are more complicated than the facade. She also maintains that it's important to understand why a woman may not be feeling beautiful and why she is sitting in her office. As Dr. Leduc explains, "My approach is predictive and preventive, which is why I want to know as much as I can about my patients. We discuss everything, including sex. Sex is very important. Nothing is taboo. Women need to talk, and they know nothing ever leaves this room."

She will often refer patients to a team of experts she has carefully assembled. She may suggest an appointment with a sports coach, a yoga teacher, a psychologist, a hypnotist, a nutritionist, a sexologist, a plastic surgeon, or an orthodontist, for example. She is also a fervent believer in meditation. "I don't think you can separate beauty and well-being," she says. She also speaks perfect English.

FRENCH PHARMACY FINDS

Whenever I think about beauty and skin care, I think about my previously mentioned pharmacist friend, Dr. Christine Salort, the mother of three teenagers and an advocate for anything one can do to promote healthy living, which in her case is a strict adherence to all that is natural, including fruits and vegetables from local farmers, home cooking, running in the forest with her dog, a glass of wine, and only care and beauty products with natural ingredients when possible. "Sometimes it's a challenge finding ingredients in beauty products that are 100 percent *bio*," she says. "In some cases, I take my essential oils and make my own products." *Bio* means originating from organic agriculture sources, which are strictly controlled by the French government.

Read on and you'll see some of Christine's essential oil recommendations for everything from dry skin to relaxing. She "prescribed" and made one recipe in particular just for me and put it in a sweet little blue bottle with a dropper top that allows me to use the precise amount and no more.

For Frenchwomen of all ages—because they learned how to take very good care of their skin as little girls from their mothers and grandmothers—meticulous skin care, which takes a certain amount of dedication, allows them to apply their makeup in about five minutes or less.

Christine is adamant about passing down good habits to her twin daughters, who have the great good fortune to have a mother who has every imaginable French product at her fingertips in her pharmacy. Her girls are plagued with acne, and Christine's approach is one all French mothers follow: She first took them to her dermatologist and then showed them how to treat the problem. She cautioned them against the impulse to use cover-up products and finally convinced them to heed her counsel.

She gave each girl her own supply of products. Included in their goody bags were three serious acne-treatment products from the Avène collection and two surprises from Roger & Gallet:

1) *Avène Cleanance Gel Nettoyant (a cleansing gel)*
2) *Avène Cleanance Mask Masque-Gommage (a mask and scrub)*
3) *Avène Cleanance Mat Lotion Matifiante (mattifying lotion)*
4) *Roger & Gallet Fleur de Figuier hand-and-nail cream*
5) *Roger & Gallet Rose hand-and-nail cream*

I often slip one of Roger & Gallet's hand and nail–cream tubes into gifts (they make sweet Christmas stocking stuffers). My favorites are the exquisite Gingembre Rouge (red ginger) or Fleur d'Osmanthus, which smells like apricots.

While we're on the subject of acne, even big girls get the occasional breakout. For those annoying problems, Christine recommends Avène TriAcnéal Expert, an emulsion in a pump.

You see, when girls begin taking care of their skin early on, they save time on the other end of the beauty spectrum as women. Imagine jumping out of bed in the morning, rinsing your face, applying a serum (many beauty experts recommend using a serum every day) and moisturizer with built-in SPF, having breakfast, then dressing and applying makeup in less than ten minutes because your skin is radiant.

You probably know that in every interview, whether with a friend or a beauty professional—including doctors—I asked them to tell me some of their favorite products. Sharing is caring, *n'est-ce pas*?

Dr. Leduc told me she is addicted to Biologique Recherche products, particularly Lotion P50, which is much more than a lotion. It's an exfoliating product with lactic and salicylic acids, which not only exfoliate, but also hydrate and balance the skin's pH. "The only problem with the product is that it smells terrible," she says.

Another of her favorites, which she uses almost every night, is Pigmentclar Serum from La Roche-Posay. It is made for dull complexions that may also have dark spots. She applies the serum with small pinching, tapping movements. "That way, I stimulate blood circulation and it works even better," she says.

I specifically chose my dermatologist, Dr. Valérie Gallais, because she understands the psychological importance of beauty to women of all ages.

Valérie (we are on a first-name basis now) usually has a new product recommendation for me. This year, it was Filorga's Optim-Eyes to help alleviate small lines, under-eye bags, and shadows. She told me to keep it in the refrigerator to boost the effect.

To get the optimal benefits from our beauty conversation, I always arrive with a list of questions. My appointments with her are a great treat; I leave her office feeling positive, clutching my Retin-A prescription, and a little bag of new products to try. How much fun is that?

THE MIND-BODY CONNECTION

As we've seen, Frenchwomen know that inner happiness is critical to outer beauty, and they make their own happiness a priority. Sometimes the best beauty secrets are to slow down and break away from the stressful cacophony of our phones and computers. More and more French doctors are recommending meditation, and recently my doctor suggested I try hypnosis to help me be more calm and mindful. Yes, I realize the word *mindful* is becoming a cliché, but I'm making a concerted effort to be more aware of living in the moment, and hypnosis has helped.

Dior's Mathilde Favier ensures a happy start to her days by beginning her mornings slowly and calmly, which she believes contributes to her general feeling of well-being. "I get out of bed between 6:45 and 7:00, have a breakfast of black coffee, pomegranate seeds, and a smoothie with a base of cold soy milk," she says. "In my world, I get up free. I do not look at my phone or my e-mails first thing in the morning. I enjoy my time, have my breakfast, look outside to see what the weather is like, open my closet, and decide what I would like to wear. Then I do ultra-quick makeup, mostly my eyes, basically nothing with my hair, and I'm pretty much out the door in less than an hour."

Removing the pressure and stress of thinking about potential problems delivered in electronic messages before we have enjoyed the first moments after waking certainly must be a beauty-enhancing trick. What could be more positive than beginning the day in your own little bubble?

My artist friend, Edith, meditates in the morning before she starts her day with tea, a plain soy yogurt, and toasted whole-grain cereal bread with honey or one of her homemade, no-sugar-added jams.

The notion of starting the day slowly and ending it similarly, by enjoying an evening toilette with fragrant products and then slipping into a beautiful bed dressed in crisp, fresh sheets, can enhance the best beauty treatment of all: a good night's sleep. All of the appropriate serums and creams are applied before tucking in because, after all, we might as well be "working" while we sleep and then wake to the results.

At least once each week, I luxuriate in a serious soak with add-ons like restorative herbs in the bathwater, masks on both my hair and face, scented candles, tea, and Édith Piaf on my stereo speaker, so that I can have a rejuvenating cry if I wish. It is tranquil and relaxing.

Alexandra Bertin, director of the Clarins spa at the Hotel Molitor in Paris, sees her spa as an escape from the energy-depleting tensions of the world. "I think we are under constant pressure in both our professional and personal lives," she says. "I'm convinced it's essential that we find restorative moments. It could mean meditation for some, walking in a forest, communing with nature, or having a massage in a spa.

"The important thing is that we reconnect with what is true and authentic and listen to what we need both physically and psychologically. A massage on its own makes us feel well and can relieve stress and sore muscles, but it must always be part of a deeper way of looking at our lives and how we want to live in a joyful way."

Alexandra is a proponent of "sophrology," a philosophy that scientifically addresses mental and physical well-being. Sophrology is fundamentally the study of the consciousness in harmony with the body. It consists of a series of easy-to-perform mind and body exercises that lead to a healthy, relaxed, calm, alert mind. The exercises are referred to as "dynamic relaxation."

Alexandra likes combining the beauty treatments of a spa with more profound sophrology classes that allow one to precisely explore the ways and means to achieve a focused and fulfilling life.

My hairstylist, Michelle, took sophrology lessons for years, practices exercises at home, and occasionally goes back to her teacher when she thinks she needs a refresher course. She says the exercises help her release not only tension, but also negative feelings about people and situations.

The rosewater I spray on my face after my makeup— or simply for a morning wake-up—is in a deep blue bottle

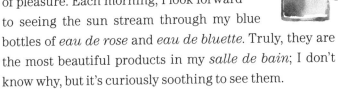

that sits on my bathroom windowsill. It is as basic as one can get in the category of beauty, but sublime in the broad definition of pleasure. Each morning, I look forward to seeing the sun stream through my blue bottles of *eau de rose* and *eau de bluette*. Truly, they are the most beautiful products in my *salle de bain*; I don't know why, but it's curiously soothing to see them.

OUR SKIN, DECADE BY DECADE AND THROUGHOUT THE YEAR

Like most of us, after trial and error and professional advice, Frenchwomen have their favorite products that work for their particular needs and specific enjoyment. At the same time, they understand that the formulas they were using at twenty, thirty, forty, fifty, and beyond need to evolve as their skin changes. Depending upon the seasons, treatments should be different to produce the best results. The logic is obvious: skin reacts differently to steamy days and frigid temperatures.

During my weeklong retreat at Les Prés d'Eugénie in the Landes region of France, I spent many hours in the *ferme thermale* relishing the ultra-luxurious spa treatments in the natural thermal waters of Eugénie les Bains. While there, I interviewed aesthetician Cécile Ledru, the director of the thermal spa and an expert on the Sisley products on offer. I asked her to break down how we should take care of our skin by the decade, and this is what she told me:

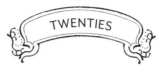

Use a rich soap, "because young women tend to like soaps, and the pharmacy has many that are kind to the skin with cold creams and other nonirritating oils. A micellar water is perfect for cleaning the face at all ages. Use appropriate day and night creams, the day having SPF built into the formula that corresponds to the seasons and sun exposure."

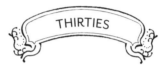

"Add an eye cream, and cleanse with a mild lotion or micellar water. Exfoliate once a week and use an appropriate mask each week."

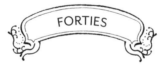

"Now is the time to get more serious. Add richer moisturizers to the routine with antioxidants, hyaluronic acid, and vitamin C. (Discuss with a dermatologist or an aesthetician.) Twice each year at the change of the seasons, do an antiaging serum treatment. Continue with once-a-week masks and exfoliation. Starting now and continuing through the decades, the masks should be *anti-rides* (anti-wrinkle)."

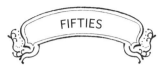

FIFTIES

"*Really* get serious now, and check with a professional to see if more *performant* products are necessary. From the forties to the fifties is an important transitional period for the skin. Menopause often requires skin care changes. Continue with masks, exfoliation, serums, and especially rich night creams."

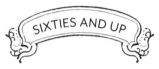

SIXTIES AND UP

"Check in with your dermatologist, but basically treatments tend to be similar from the fifties to the sixties and after."

Cécile is a huge advocate for vitamins A, C, and E in skin-care products. She also loves coconut oil, which she uses "on everything: hair, body, face, nails, feet, and hands. It's brilliant," she says. "Before I go to bed, I slather my feet with coconut oil, cover them with plastic wrap, and slip on socks. In the morning, I slough off the dead skin in the shower, and my feet are soft and smooth."

Cécile lived in Brazil before France, and during those years, she made her own beauty products with the resources at hand. She used fine sugar and lemon as a scrub on her face and lips. For a mask, she used honey that she applied generously on her face, massaging it into her skin until it turned white, then rinsing thoroughly. She said the results were "*fantastique.*"

MORE ADVICE: "Change masks according to the seasons. You will not need the same one in summer as in fall and winter," she says. "Don't use the same products all the time. Our skin gets tired of the same things, even though we may like them. Take a break and then come back to a product you like." Dr. Gallais, for example, has been emphasizing the change-it-up routine for years.

FROM WITHIN

When I ask Frenchwomen about beauty, without exception they say, "True beauty comes from within." Trite? Clichéd? I don't think so.

The other day, while sitting for hours having my hair *balayaged*, I read an article in a French magazine wherein women of all ages discussed style and beauty. One of the women, in her late forties, said that if the most beautiful woman in the world were rude, aggressive, and condescending, "suddenly she would be lessbeautiful." The other women in the article agreed.

> "Nature gives you the face you have at twenty. Life shapes the face you have at thirty. But at fifty, you get the face you deserve."
>
> —COCO CHANEL

When I was young, I took piano lessons for many years and absolutely loved my piano teacher, who I often referred to as "the beautiful Miss Frank." Apparently she was not a great beauty, but I liked her so much that I saw her as beautiful.

Could it be possible that kindness, charm, intelligence, generosity, and warmth are the true secrets to beauty? (Yes, we want to do the best we can with our natural resources and we know that with a little help from a dermatologist and our products we'll look and feel better, but life marches on and it behooves us to find beauty inside and out to have *la joie de vivre*. And I guarantee what comes from within will be reflected on your face.)

MAKEUP: ADVICE FROM THE EXPERTS

Once our skin is radiant and the canvas is prepared, the fine art of makeup becomes a breeze. The experts always have well-tested techniques to help us appear more beautiful and accomplish the ultimate goal of looking fresh and natural. After a certain age, the last result we want from our artifice is to have it *look* like artifice.

Before starting her own cosmetics line, By Terry, in 1998, the very beautiful Terry de Gunzburg worked for fifteen years creating revolutionary products for Yves Saint Laurent. It was there that she invented the iconic Touche Éclat, a magic-wand "pen"—actually a soft, strategically formed brush—that brightens and perfects the complexion while both highlighting and covering imperfections without adding any glittery effects.

You have already met Terry in other chapters, so now let me tell you some of her makeup advice for women of a certain age:

   ❧ "What I tend to see is too much or not enough makeup."

- ❧ "My number one rule is less is more. Women need to learn to work a small amount of foundation into their skin to make it look natural."
- ❧ "A brush is the best way to apply foundation, and a woman needs very little when it is worked into the skin well. It should become so invisible that it appears to be her natural complexion."
- ❧ "Before you apply foundation, begin with a color-correcting primer, which will brighten the skin, reduce dark spots, and take out redness in order to prepare an even base."
- ❧ "It's important for a woman's well-being and self-esteem to have a manicure, wear perfume, and pay attention to unseen details like well-cared-for feet and pretty lingerie."
- ❧ If you're in a bad mood, put on some lipstick. It totally changes your attitude and forces you to smile."

Eric Antoniotti, the international artistic and training director for Clarins, is one of my favorite people. He is down-to-earth and, best of all, irreverently funny. If you are familiar with my last book, you met him in the beauty chapter. This time, we met for coffee and had a grand time gossiping and talking about what changes he has observed on the beauty scene since we last spoke. This is what he told me:

- ❧ "Even since the last time we talked about beauty, the textures of makeup products have improved. They make the skin look brighter, discreetly hide imperfections, and make the complexion appear

'glow-y' without glitter. It's a sort of extremely
flattering spotlight effect."

✧ "Do I need to say this? Less is more. Always."

✧ "I like a color-correcting cream in a Champagne
tone to build upon."

✧ "Serums are of the utmost importance. Every
woman needs a serum. She should ask for
professional advice in choosing which one would
be best for her. There are serums that are 'tensers,'
others that lift a bit, and some that brighten and
clarify. It's not always easy to find the right one, so ask."

✧ "I like to mix primer with foundation. You
need very little product, and you apply
it with a purpose-made brush so, like
painting, you can make long strokes,
thus drawing out the product for fine,
almost invisible coverage."

✧ "Rose blushes work for every woman. They give
freshness and radiance."

✧ "When finished applying makeup, gently pat, pat,
pat the face to 'set' the products with your warm,
clean hands."

✧ "I can never emphasize how important the brows
are. I always use a brow kit that has two to three
different powders so that I can make a custom color
each time."

✧ "When applying makeup, never have the light over
your head because it creates shadows. The best
place is sitting in front of a source of natural light."

- "Always remember to brush through lashes after applying mascara. There is nothing quite as aging as seeing clumpy lashes."
- "Forget about orangey or fuchsia lip colors. When choosing a natural color for everyday, think about nudes that are not too pink or too beige. The best color for everyone is one or two shades darker than the real color of the lips."
- "One trick I like is to have a woman hold up a tube of lipstick, look into a mirror, and see if the color 'speaks' to her, then try to get a sample. Instinct counts."
- "Frenchwomen are not into contouring with dark powders because it's not natural; they prefer highlighting, not shadows."
- "Honestly, once a woman learns how to do her makeup in the best way for her needs, it takes five minutes or less to apply her everyday routine."

Before becoming the artistic director of Guerlain and creating exceptional fragrances for the perfume house, Sylvaine Delacourte was a makeup artist. When I discovered that detail in her beauty résumé, I brought out my list of beauty questions, and she graciously said:

- "Always do a five-to-ten-minute mask, rinse, and then spray the face with icy-cold water to prepare a naturally pretty tint before applying makeup. It changes everything."
- "Next, apply a day cream by pressing on the skin from the center toward the exterior of the face with

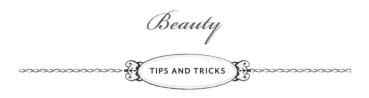

Beauty

Here are some of my favorite tips that I've picked up over the years from department-store makeup counters, Sephora, French friends, and interviews:

- A flesh-colored pencil traced into the water line of the eye opens up the eye.

- To make lips appear fuller, dot a tiny bit of highlighter into your cupid's bow.

- For those with naturally thin lips or lips that have become thinner with age (I know, I know ...), avoid matte lipsticks and apply lipstick with a brush. First, lightly outline the lips with the same color or, even better, a colorless liner (it's impossible to make a messy mistake in the application). Do not line as if you were doing an outline on a drawing—keep it soft and natural to hold lipstick inside the lips while lightly defining them.

- After applying lipstick, pat the lips with your ring finger to "soften" the look, then apply a dab of gloss in the top and bottom center of the lips.

- Vitamin C helps brighten complexions.

- Wash all makeup brushes at least once each week. You can use shampoo or products specifically made for the job.

- Toss mascara after three to four months.

- Our eyelashes often become sparse with age. To create your own trompe l'oeil effect, take a brown or black eye pencil and dot, dot, dot at the roots of the lashes, which makes it seem as if lashes are thicker. Then, of course, curl lashes with the best of the best from Shu Uemura and apply a volumizing mascara.

- Cream blushes are better for older skin because they melt into the complexion and appear natural, whereas powders can cake, sit on top of the skin, and sink into wrinkles.

- Terry de Gunzburg has a brilliant concealer in her By Terry line, Touche Veloutée, which I think is better than the original Touché Eclat.

your fingertips. By doing this, you're stimulating circulation, bringing blood to the surface."

- "Mix your foundation with a gel serum to lift and fix the skin."
- "Apply foundation with a brush for a clean finish without product buildup."

GOOD HAIR DAYS

Although I did no in-depth reporting on hair for this book (see my first book, *Forever Chic,* for more on Frenchwomen's tips for beautiful hair), let me review a few essentials so that hair care will also fall into the fast-and-easy column. Once again, preparation sets the stage: a superb cut truly takes into account one's type of hair and the amount of patience one has with fussing. I, for example, have no patience for fussing. As I sit here in front of my computer, my almost-shoulder-length hair is in a ponytail.

To color or not to color is an intimately personal decision. If I had gorgeous gray or white hair, I would go natural. I don't. My formerly—*way* formerly—blonde hair is now some base color that could best be described as watered-down mud. Therefore, I spend a fortune on *balayage*, but it's my great luxury and it makes me extremely happy.

Below are a few quick reminders to keep your hair shiny and healthy that I reviewed with hairstylists Michelle, who does my color, and Estelle, who does my cut. Michelle is in the country not far from us; Estelle, who I have followed from salon to salon for more than fifteen years, is in Paris.

I would follow her to the North Pole for one of her cuts. This is what they told me:

- "Above all else, you want your hair to 'move,' otherwise it's aging—a little depressing," Estelle says. "The last thing a woman should want is hair that looks fixed. If it doesn't look natural, it's not flattering."
- Twice-per-week shampoos are the maximum necessary. Alternate shampoo products. I alternate between Kérastase Reflection Bain Chromatique and Christophe Robin's Crème Lavante, which is a cleansing mask.
- Hair looks best the day after and the day after that of a shampoo.
- Forget about products, products, products. If you want a smooth finish, just the slightest light hair spray will keep flyaways tamed.
- Both recommend buying basic products: shampoos, instant conditioners, and deep conditioners or masks from hair salons because, they say, the brands are more concentrated, more *performant* (that is, they work better), and therefore you will need much less.
- Michelle recommends sleeping in a deep-conditioning hair mask beneath a shower cap once a month.
- Christophe Robin is one of the world's most famous colorists, and he understands the importance of taking extremely good care of our hair, whether colored or not. Another of my favorite products

from his line is Brume Volume Naturel à l'Eau de Rose, a volumizing mist with rosewater that is sprayed on damp, just-shampooed hair at the roots and all the way down to the ends. The *eau de rose* is sublime.

- I regularly use Christophe Robin's Huile à Lavande moisturizing hair oil with lavender, and his Masque Fixateur de Couleur au Germe de Blé, a color-fixing mask with wheat germ. (He gave me these products when I interviewed him for my last book, and I've been buying them ever since.)

- Occasionally, once or twice each month before a shampoo, I warm an oil, Moroccan, argan, or jojoba, in the palm of my hands and apply to my hair, paying particular attention to the ends. I alternate this with Christophe Robin's lavender oil. Christophe recommended this trick, and Michelle and Estelle agree. In France, Moroccan argan oil is considered to be liquid gold, not for its price but because it is rich, easily absorbed, and not too greasy and can be used on every inch of the body. It works wonders on all our stubborn dry-skin areas, from elbows to feet and ankles. A little goes a long way.

- Dry shampoo can be a true beauty boon when there is no time to shampoo and you just need to tidy up a bit at the roots. The best brand is Klorane, and just a couple of whooshes, gently massaged into the scalp with a light brushing, do the trick. Some Frenchwomen use dry shampoos as volume

boosters. Rumor has it that that's how Karl
Lagerfeld keeps his hair powdery white.

Another cult product for the hair is a confidential mix of botanical oils in Leonor Greyl's Huile Secret de Beauté, which can also be used on the body, although I don't know anyone who does. (An appealing aspect to the product is that, in a global world where mega-conglomerates own more brands than most of us imagine, the Leonor Greyl line continues to be a family-owned business, now run by Caroline Greyl, daughter of Leonor.)

Our hair and bodies do love rich oils, and there are scores of them in a vast range of prices. Leonor Greyl oil is expensive, but if pricey products do not fit into your budget, argan oil, bought from a health-food store, most definitely will.

Because my hair is almost shoulder-length, thick, and slightly wavy, I use a Wet Brush (it's not a brush that is wet, but rather a brand of hairbrush that I use— I bought another one for my granddaughter whose hair is a mass of curls) to minimize the torture of inevitable tangles.

Once again, most of the women of a certain age I interviewed preferred hairstyles no longer than just skimming the shoulders or even shorter. Michelle and Estelle felt that the shoulder length was not flattering on women after a certain age, yet many women of a certain age disagree.

Chanel's Marie-Louise de Clermont-Tonnerre agreed about after-a-certain-age haircuts. She cut her hair a few years ago to a shorter bob and feels that it's the best choice;

she maintains that shorter hair is more flattering for a mature face.

When I first interviewed Dior's Mathilde Favier, who is in her forties, she had thick, eyebrow-skimming bangs and a simple, chin-length blunt cut. The next time I saw her, she had a gamine pixie that changed absolutely everything about her look. The new style had a magic effect on her allure. It's proof, once again, that finding the haircut that reflects and enhances one's personality is a beauty boon.

J'ADORE LE PARFUM

It would be impossible to write about beauty and Frenchwomen of a certain age without including fragrance. Perfume is sensual, profoundly personal, evocative, and magical. Perfume is an extension of our personality and our style. It creates lasting memories, and it's a way to communicate something lovely without saying a word. As you can see, I adore perfume. I turned to two women deeply immersed in the creation of luscious scents to talk about their passion.

Sylvaine Delacourte, who after 180 years of patriarchic perfume creation in the legendary Guerlain maison became the first female "nose" to imagine fragrances of unforgettable elegance and beauty. Today, she continues in the role of consultant to the revered perfumer, now owned by LVMH, while at the same time venturing out under her own name with a collection of extraordinary musk-based eau de parfums.

I had always thought of musk as a dark, deeply sultry essence, but in our interview Sylvaine explains—and proves—that musk is far more interesting, versatile, and complex.

Sylvaine has blended irises from Tuscany, roses from Bulgaria, tonka beans from Venezuela, and spices from Kerala, India, into her perfumes. All are named after women, although she says men as well as women are drawn to the scents.

Sylvaine also believes that it's unimaginable to separate fragrance from *l'art de vivre*. "Perfume is emotion," she says. "It must make a woman feel something, otherwise it has no appeal. One must never forget that it is the woman who 'personalizes' a perfume, as it becomes her signature with her unique skin mingling with the ingredients."

In our interview over tea at the Hôtel Lancaster in Paris, she describes how she imagines perfume in her mind before she sets out to construct a fragrance. She calls herself an "olfactive profiler." One of her talents is conjuring custom *sur mesure* perfume, tailored specifically for one woman. In order to create the singular fragrance, she interviews the lucky woman, asks her myriad questions, and then goes to work mixing her olfactory translation of what she was told. When the woman finds the ultimate recipe that reflects who she is, Sylvaine gives her the recipe that will never be used for anyone else in the world.

Such a creation has a hefty price tag: a unique perfume can ring in at about $55,000 for two liters in an exquisite Baccarat bottle. But wouldn't it be marvelous to have a signature perfume become part of a family's history, the formula passed on for generations?

Some of Sylvaine's special secrets include:

- You can keep an unopened perfume in the refrigerator for up to ten years. (Now, I imagine this would be if you have fallen madly in love with a fragrance and worry that one day it might be discontinued; you're planning for the future.)
- Contrary to what we've heard, the color of our skin has nothing to do with how a perfume smells, it's far more complex than that.
- We tend to be drawn, unknowingly, to our "olfactive patrimony" when choosing a perfume. Buried in our subconscious are olfactive memories that are exhibited in certain notes in the formula, like grass or our grand-mother's perfume or a flower garden from our childhood.
- From time to time, spray your eau de toilette on your sheets.
- Keep a small, travel-size refill of your fragrance in your purse at all times. You never know.
- Put a few drops of your perfume in a neutral body cream.
- You can replace a perfume product for a friend or give him or her another item in the line like soap, bath gel, or lotion, but fragrance is such a personal extension of one's personality that it's best not to guess what he or she might like.
- Always test a new fragrance for a week; samples will last at least that long. See if you like it as much as you did

when you tried it at the perfumer and wait to see how those close to you react to your new find.

A few days before meeting Sylvaine, I had tea with Virginie Roux, whose family has supplied flowers for generations to some of the world's most prestigious perfume houses. In 1998, Virginie and her husband, Antoine, founded Au Pays de la Fleur d'Oranger from, as they proclaimed, "a shared passion of the regional flowers of Grasse and fragrances that have molded their Provence landscape and families for generations." The couple grew up surrounded by the romantic, comforting scents of bitter orange and *Rosa centifolia* (the cabbage or May rose), flowers which have become the house's statement fragrances. They hired an experienced and creative nose, Jean-Claude Gigodot, to bring their vision to life with a collection of luxe fragrances. And now for a few special secrets from Virginie:

- Because of one's skin and hormonal makeup, a perfume can be "mute." In other words, it doesn't work. It evokes no pleasure or emotion.
- When trying a new perfume on the wrists, never rub the wrists together. The friction breaks down the molecules of a formula and gives a false reading of the fragrance.
- When trying several perfumes, "clear the palette" between samplings at a perfume counter by taking a deep breath on another part of the skin. It's impossible to be discerning among the inhalations of several bouquets.
- Never put on too much perfume. It's always better to reapply throughout the day.

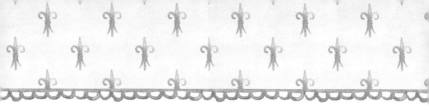

The Nine Best Spots
TO APPLY PERFUME

Here are nine strategic areas to anoint, according to Sylvaine:

- The roots of the hair on the back of the neck.

- The wrists, but not too close to the hands so that it's not washed away.

- Inside the elbows.

- Between the breasts.

- The navel.

- Your hair—spray it on your hairbrush.

- Behind the knees (so people seated can appreciate your fragrance as you breeze by).

- On your clothes, particularly scarves and sweaters.

- A piece of cotton sprayed with perfume and slipped into your bra.

> *"Apply perfume where you want to be kissed."*
>
> —COCO CHANEL

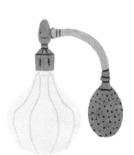

- ❧ Remember that perfume is a language.
- ❧ Women are chameleons, and more than ever they like to change their fragrances and have a few in rotation depending upon mood and the seasons.
- ❧ Fragrance can be a mask that perhaps we can hide behind.

PERFUME, HISTORICALLY SPEAKING

I don't know about you, but I love trivia. For that reason, I thought I would share a few perfume trifles with you from a couple of my favorite history books:

- ❧ Centuries ago, when bathing was not of primary importance and indoor plumbing had yet to be invented, perfume was a useful means to smell good when perhaps you didn't.
- ❧ Louis XV adored perfume to the point where his court became known as *La Cour Parfumée*. His mistress, Madame de Pompadour, had refinement and a penchant toward the lovely and the extravagant and became a patron to perfumers.
- ❧ During this period, not only did the unwashed apply perfume to their bodies, they also applied it to their clothes and even their furniture.
- ❧ Marie Antoinette's passion for flowers throughout the rooms in Versailles was responsible for captivating fragrances wafting through the air to the great pleasure of the court and visitors.
- ❧ Today, most women opt for eau de parfum or eau de toilette, with aromatic oil concentrations of about 15 and 10 percent, respectively. Perfume, ever

considered a luxury, has a concentration of about 25 to 30 percent, and the weakest of the collection of fragrances, eau de cologne, has approximately a 3 percent concentration. *Silage,* a new word for me (and I've been writing about perfume for decades) means the staying power of a fragrance once we apply it to our bodies. It's the lingering scent that we leave in the air, but it apparently has nothing to do with the amount of perfume we apply. It's probably another aspect of the mystery of perfume.

- The five most popular perfumes in the world, in ascending order, are: L'Air du Temps by Nina Ricci; Opium by Yves Saint Laurent; Shalimar by Guerlain; Joy by Jean Patou; and Chanel No. 5, the number one fragrance of all time. I've worn all but Shalimar, which I don't like on me, and Joy, which my best childhood friend has worn for as long as I can remember (which means she *owns* it). For me, L'Air du Temps is exquisite and was my first grown-up perfume. I had every product in the line, from soap and bath powder to body lotion and real perfume. It's sublime.

- The sweet success of Chanel No. 5 is a story of serendipity. Coco Chanel was asked to choose from a lineup of banal bottles, marked only with numbers, to be her first perfume. By chance she chose bottle number five because that was her lucky number. Then the perfume, the first to have a "recipe" that included several ingredients, was launched on May 5, 1921—the fifth day of the fifth month.

✧ The house of Dior introduced its first fragrance, Miss Dior, in 1947, dedicated to Christian Dior's sister. Instead of naming the perfume Mademoiselle Dior, Monsieur Dior chose *Miss* because he was a devout Anglophile.

✧ Rose and jasmine are the most commonly used scents in perfume, and apparently almost every perfume in the world contains one or both. They are appreciated for their gorgeous aromas, of course, but also because the essences are easy to extract from the plants.

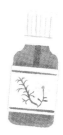

THE BEAUTY OF ESSENTIAL OILS

My pharmacist, Dr. Christine Salort, also has a passion for essential oils. She has studied them for years and devoted an inordinate amount of shelf space to them in her pharmacy; she is a veritable wizard when it comes to combining the essences. Although opinion is divided on the efficacy of essential oils, I include here some of her favorite recipes. As always, consult your doctor first:

✧ FOR MORE PHYSICAL ENERGY: A combination of half Scotch pine oil and half spruce oil. Warm eight drops in the palms of the hands and gently rub on the lower back just above the kidneys. Use for two to three weeks.

✧ FOR MORALE AND PSYCHOLOGICAL BOOST: Breathe in bergamot, peppermint, or ylang-ylang oil.

✧ TO RELAX: Try lavender, bitter orange, or sweet orange oil. For children, try mandarin oil before bedtime.

Apply to the pulse points as well as the bottom of the feet. Then breathe deeply.

- TO SLEEP: Use ravensara oil (it has a light eucalyptus fragrance), which is known for its antidepressant and anti-stress benefits; also try sweet almond and lavender. Apply either down the spinal cord or on the bottoms of the feet.
- FOR A HANGOVER: Use a drop each of rosemary, lemon, and peppermint on a small sugar cube. Consume quickly.
- FOR CELLULITE AND DRY SKIN: Try avocado oil massaged onto the affected areas.
- FOR PSORIASIS: Use borage oil gently rubbed onto the skin. "Borage has many uses, from an anti-stress remedy to relieving rheumatoid arthritis pain," Christine says.
- FOR GENERAL FATIGUE: Rub wheat germ oil onto the skin.
- FOR EXTRA-DRY SKIN: Massage macadamia nut oil generously onto the body.
- FOR DARK, PUFFY EYES: Rub two drops of calophyllum oil between your index fingers and gently tap and massage beneath the eyes.

During one of my visits to say hello to Christine, I complained that my skin wasn't looking or feeling good, and was blotchy, red, and dull. She told me I was doing too much, using too many treatment products too often, and that my poor face needed a rest. She then said she had just the prescription to get me back to normal, and I should come back tomorrow.

The next day, she handed over a lovely little blue bottle filled with a mélange of essential oils she had made just for me. "It's full of antioxidants and fatty acids, with lots of nourishing properties. You'll see a difference in about ten days," she said. Clearly I needed her concoction, because the oil had been totally absorbed before I climbed into bed and only the delectable fragrance remained, which I think helped me fall asleep. Christine says that is a "side benefit" of the treatment.

I asked her for the recipe so I could share it with you. All of the ingredients are *bio,* she emphasizes. The first three are vegetal oils, and the remaining five are essential oils. Vegetal oils act as "carriers" for the essential oils to be used on the body. I did the conversion from metric, and one milliliter is one-fifth of a teaspoon—not so easy to measure.

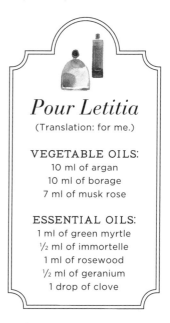

Pour Letitia

(Translation: for me.)

VEGETABLE OILS:
10 ml of argan
10 ml of borage
7 ml of musk rose

ESSENTIAL OILS:
1 ml of green myrtle
½ ml of immortelle
1 ml of rosewood
½ ml of geranium
1 drop of clove

Squeeze and fill the dropper, squirt the oils into your clean hands, rub lightly until the liquid is warm, then pat your face and go to bed.

A WORD OF CAUTION: While out and about doing interviews and sampling everything from food and wine to beauty and treatment products, I discovered, to my great surprise, that I was highly allergic to a luxury brand of cosmetics that boast their natural ingredients. The reaction was instant. My face turned blazing red, and my skin burned so much that I almost cried. Lots of cool water and an ice pack brought everything back to normal in a couple of hours. This is the first time I have ever had a bad reaction to a product. All of this being said, I want to caution you that although essential oils are natural, you should consult your doctor and do a test before committing.

SOME OF MY FAVORITE PRODUCTS

I always follow the counsel of my dermatologist, Dr. Valérie Gallais, with diligence and delight, and her recommendation is to vary the use of treatment products. That translates into using one until it runs out and replacing it with another and then going back to the first. Maybe—if I can't resist—I'll try something new.

Below is a list of my favorite and most *performant* products by category. Some have never changed because I can't break up our meaningful relationship—for all the right reasons. Then I've added a number of new entries. All come recommended by my coterie of experts; I have never bought a treatment product on impulse. And of course I have no financial benefit from any product I mention and only tell you about those that I have used at the recommendation of doctors or my pharmacist friend. If I don't like a product, find it doesn't live up to its promises, or I have an allergic reaction, I don't mention them. As always, my try-before-you-buy counsel, taking advantage of samples, is the only way to find out what works for you, and in consultation with your dermatologist.

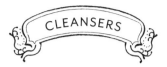

CLEANSERS

- Bioderma ABCDerm H2O Solution Micellaire
- Vichy Pureté Thermale 3-in-1 One Step Cleanser
- La Roche-Posay Effaclar Deep Cleansing Foaming Cream
- Nuxe Bio Beauté Lotion-Soin Détox, Anti-Pollution et Éclat
- Roger & Gallet Le Soin Aura Mirabilis Masque
  Extra-Fin Démaquillant *(a makeup remover)*

Christine introduced me to this last product, which is both a makeup remover and a mask. It is so much fun to use and full of natural ingredients, and it smells wonderful in the most subtle way. It goes on as a sort of thick gel, which turns into a lotion while you massage. Then you rinse it away, and skin looks refreshed. It can also be left on the face as a mask. I don't understand it, but I see the results.

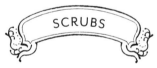

SCRUBS

- Nuxe Gentle Exfoliating Gel with Rose Petals
- La Roche-Posay Gommage Surfin Physiologique
- Dermaceutic Laboratoire Foamer 15 Exfoliating Cleansing
  Foam *(It's serious, with 15 percent glycolic acid, and may not be tolerated by very sensitive skin. I love it, but I use it only once per week. It was recommended by Dr. Gallais.)*

NOTE: When it comes to exfoliating, don't overdo it. Apply the gentlest touch to the massages that accompany the procedure and always remember to follow with moisturizer. Some dermatologists recommend less exfoliation in the summer so as not to make the skin more fragile.

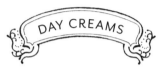

- Eucerin Hyaluron-Filler Day SPF15. *The addition of sun protection is new to the hyaluronic-acid formula.*
- Filorga Hydra-Filler Pro-Youth Moisturizer
- La Roche-Posay Redermic R Corrective UV SPF 30 with retinol
- La Roche-Posay Redermic C for normal to combination skin.

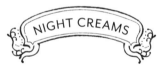

- Eucerin Hyaluron-Filler Night
- Filorga Nutri-Filler
- Christine's *Pour Letitia* special, *once-a-week deep treatment*

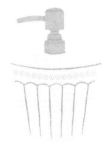

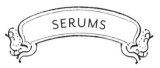

SERUMS

- Filorga Hydra-Hyal Intensive Hydrating Plumping Concentrate *(can be used alone or with night and day creams)*
- Auriga International Flavo-C Forte
- Lierac Premium Sérum Régénérant
- Roger & Gallet Le Soin Aura Mirabilis Double-Extrait *(This was a present from Christine because she just bought a new range from Roger & Gallet for her pharmacy. It is to be used with the Roger & Gallet mask. It smells like a summer garden.)*

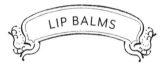

LIP BALMS

- Nuxe Baume Lèvres Ultra-Nourrissant Rêve de Miel
- Labello Soin des Lèvres
- Avène Care for Sensitive Lips
- Garnier Ultra Doux Trésors de Miel

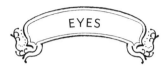

EYES

- Filorga Optim-Eyes Eye Contour *(This is one of the latest recommendations from Dr. Gallais. It is excellent and best kept in the refrigerator to boost the effect.)*
- Emgryolisse *(This double-action stick product brightens and smooths the contour around the eyes. It reduces dark circles and puffiness and works even better when stored in the refrigerator. Makeup artists love it.)*

BOUTONS

(pimples)

- La Roche-Posay Effaclar Duo Acne Treatment
- Prescription Retin-A

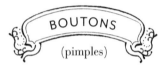

MASKS

- Avène Soothing Moisture Mask *(It's deeply hydrating, and sometimes I sleep in it.)*
- Nocibé Masque Capsules *(Each mask is a separate capsule: cranberry for éclat [brightness]; argile [clay] for purification; aloe vera for hydration; honey for nourishment; and ginger for antiaging. These are fast and fun.)*
- Payot My Payot Sleeping Pack Anti-Fatigue Sleeping Mask *(Cleanse face, apply a thin layer, change your pillowcase, and go to bed.)*

- Nuxe Crème Fraîche de Beauté Masque *(a soothing and rehydrating mask)*
- Decléor Life Radiance Flash Radiance Mask

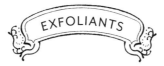

- Nuxe Body Gommage Corps Fondant with almond and orange flower petals *(I use this in combination with Nuxe body gel with the same fragrance.)*
- Linéance Gommage Intense
- Garnier Gommage Beauté Absolue
- Clarins Exfoliating Body Scrub for Smooth Skin with Bamboo Powders
- Une Olive en Provence Body Scrub with olive oil and powdered olive pits. *(This was a gift from a friend and I'm loving it.)*

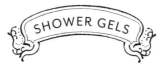

- Roger & Gallet's range of gels *is wonderful. I like all of them and change from one to another as I finish the tube.*
- Biolane Gel Lavant Surgras *is a creamy wash for babies, which I bought for my granddaughter, Ella. It has no fragrance, is extremely hydrating, and is a nice, rich alternative when skin can get dry in the winter.*

- **A-Derma,** *which my dermatologist recommended for extra-dry and irritated skin. It is more of an oil than a gel, but made for the shower. Its soothing formula is gentle enough for babies and for face and body cleansing. It is full of plants and extracts.*
- Cadum Crème Douche au Talc Surdoux et Lait d'Amandes *(This is another one of those products that families begin using with babies, and then the entire family continues using it.)*

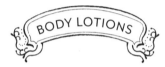
BODY LOTIONS

As you know, there are hundreds of perfumed products available, many of which echo the fragrances of our perfumes, but for this category I've chosen lotions with no, or almost no, scent. All are serious skin repairers recommended by dermatologists and pharmacists.

- Avène TriXera Nutrition Nutri-Fluid Lotion
- Avène Cold Cream Nourishing Body Lotion
- A-Derma Baume Emollient *(It is mild enough for babies, nourishes, calms irritations, and relieves itchiness from dry skin.)*
- Ducray Ictyane HD Lipid-Replenishing Anti-Irritant Balm
- Topicrem Ultra-Hydrating Long-Lasting Body Milk
- Akileïne Pieds Tres Secs *(My absolute favorite cream for extra-dry feet, recommended by medical pedicurists licensed by the state.)*

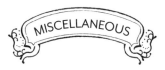

- **Sanoflore Organic Ancient Rose Floral Water** *is a natural, refreshing toner. In the summer, I keep it in the refrigerator.*

- **Avène Cicalfate Restorative Skin Cream** *(It is touted as a product to be used post-procedure but is superb for general skin repair. I always have a tube in my medicine cabinet.)*

- **Uriage Bariéderm is for the little boo-boos in life.**

- **Løv Organic Hibiscus,** *a sort of "tea" but not really, was introduced to me by my French niece, who is also a doctor and another proponent of all things natural that go in or on the body. It's an organic mix of pomegranate, hibiscus, and goji berries, reputed for their refreshing and energizing properties. (I think this could be a lovely gift for its virtues, but also because it comes in an adorable blue tin.)*

- **Biafine** *is great for little wounds and burns and adored for soothing sunburns.*

- **Homeoplasmine** *is so popular, it has its own hashtag. Its reputation for soothing chapped lips, sore noses, and little abrasions has turned it into a treatment rock star. Makeup artists like it because it leaves a matte rather than a slick surface on lips, which makes it a perfect base for lipsticks.*

- **Avène Eau Thermale,** *which goes in the refrigerator in the summer. It's impossible to live without this.*

꙳ La Roche-Posay Anthelios Ultra Light SPF6o Sunscreen

꙳ Caudalié French Kiss Lip Balm *(gives that "bitten lips" look we love)*

꙳ Caudalié Beauty Elixir *(a magic mist loved by makeup artists and me)*

꙳ Christophe Robin Antioxidant Cleansing Milk with 4 Oils and Blueberry *(refreshes my* balayage*)*

꙳ Clarins Beauty Flash Balm

ALL FOR BEAUTY

Beauty is intrinsically bound to *l'art de vivre à la française.* To this day, we continue to be intrigued by some of the dangerous products women from the past were willing to use in the name of beauty.

Marie Antoinette, it is said, took to her bed wearing gloves lined with wax, rosewater, and sweet almond oil after cleansing her face with *eau de pigeon.* And yes, the unfortunate recipe did include real pigeons.

Her favorite facial mask for a glowing complexion, according to *Vogue,* included two teaspoons of cognac, one-third cup of dry milk powder, a squeeze of lemon juice, and one egg white. Apparently some Frenchwomen continue to whip up the mask today and swear by its efficacy.

It's impossible to overemphasize the notion that beauty and pleasure are inextricably bound for a Frenchwoman. I think their *real* beauty secret is not only their loyalty to their beauty rituals, which give them appreciable results from their favorite products, but also the pleasure they take in these rituals.

Among the Frenchwomen I know, prevention and maintenance are their priorities. Their goal is to age gracefully and look the best they can. All are willing to devote the time necessary to achieve that end while having a good time in the process. It is a lesson we all could take to heart. When you feel good, you look good—simple as that.

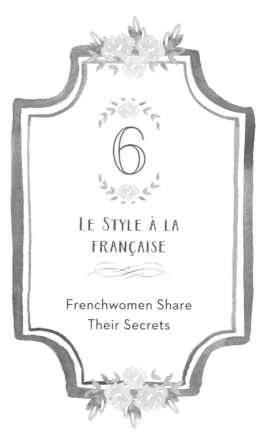

6

LE STYLE À LA FRANÇAISE

Frenchwomen Share
Their Secrets

Any conversation about *l'art de vivre à la française* would be incomplete without celebrating the internationally renowned style of Frenchwomen of a certain age.

We've all seen that such a woman oozes a confident sense of well-being when entering a room or walking down the street. She could be like the fiftysomething woman I saw the other day when My-Reason-For-Living-In-France and I had lunch in Paris.

It was early fall, and she was having lunch with three women. They were deep into that special best-friends kind of animated conversation. I couldn't take my eyes off of her. The others were well-dressed, but for me, she had the *je ne sais quoi* that set her apart. She was wearing a simple gray crewneck sweater and well-tailored gray flannel trousers. But best of all, she had on a pair of huge sparkly statement earrings, a large ring on one hand, and a wide silver cuff on the opposite wrist. Her fingernails were painted a deep red. Her dark shoulder-length hair was loose and unfussy, and it appeared she wore very little makeup.

The earrings lit up her face and moved in a swingy rhythm as she talked and laughed. It made me wonder if she were as lighthearted and warm as she appeared. At the very least, it was clear she was having a delightful time.

At the end of her lunch, she air-kissed her friends goodbye, slipped a lightweight white wool coat over her shoulders, and departed before the others. I still regret not jumping up, dashing out the door after her, telling her how chic I thought she was, and then asking her about her earrings—a missed opportunity.

That woman, whom I will never see again, made me realize how little it takes to make the simple special. It's *always* all about the details. The details could be accessories, as they were in this case, but they could also be the fit of a garment, the length of a skirt or jacket, a splash of an unexpected bright color against a neutral ensemble, the assemblage of a tone-on-tone color family, some surprising addition like a mauve coat over a navy blue outfit, or the way a large scarf is tied. The possibilities are almost infinite.

BE ORIGINAL

Mathilde Favier is one of those women whom you cannot look at without admiring her very personal style and cheerful nonchalance. The first day we met, she was wearing jeans and a gray pullover, feet bare, toenails polished, little or no makeup. She *owned* the ultra simple look. Everything about her reflects an exuberant allure—her smile, her warmth, and her intelligence. The way she dresses is an extension of her bubbly personality.

The next time I saw her, she had cut her hair into a gamine pixie. The style changed everything about her, and yet the cut *was* Mathilde. It looked like it was created just for her.

When I ask Mathilde about the subject at hand, she tells me the first rule we should all live by is to "never try to be someone other than ourselves. A woman needs to figure out who she is, stay true to herself, and take advantage of all her attributes," she says.

Time and again, I've observed and been told by Frenchwomen that they learned at an early age that there is no point or advantage in trying to emulate some supposed fashion icon who is probably dressed by a professional stylist. Mothers and grandmothers teach their descendants, both by example and explanation, that the only way to be yourself is to be different, "original," as fashion legend Diana Vreeland said. You are you. Figure out what you like about yourself and make the most of it. However, inspiration is everywhere. Observe, absorb, use the takeaways that work for you, and then make them yours.

I spent the better part of my career explaining just how to do that under headlines that cried out "This Season's Latest Trends!" As a fashion editor, I've written hundreds of stories on what's new and what's next when I returned from covering ready-to-wear collections in Milan, London, Japan, Germany, and New York, and both ready-to-wear and haute couture in Paris. And honestly, I loved every second of it. Still, when I came back to my desk from the shows, I always wrote an equal number of pieces on how to take the runway into the real world as I did on my literal reporting of what I saw on the catwalk.

The best part for me was translating some of the tricked-out costumes necessary to build excitement on a runway into wearable wardrobe pieces. Sometimes it was a color story, or an accessory or a new shape, but there was *always* a usable takeaway.

That's another reason that to this day, I still love the thick spring and fall French fashion magazines filled with all the news about what's new and now. When we learn how to look at these magazines, we can see that among the latest and greatest offerings from a current season, there are classics in the mix without fail. Maybe it's a blazer in a new fabric or color, a shirt that has a special detail that sets it apart and makes it interesting, a pair of shoes, statement earrings(!), or a great coat. I use these magazines as reference materials because, if we're looking for something—even if we don't yet know exactly what—the ideas and the tricks are there for the taking.

IT'S ALL ABOUT ATTITUDE

Let's not forget, too, that attitude, the mind-set a French-woman takes with her when dressing, is her ultimate fashion accessory.

A recent report from the J. Walter Thompson Innovation Group shows that Baby Boomer women do not define themselves by age. The report refers to this demographic as "Elastic Generation: The Female Edit," which includes women who proclaim they enjoy life more now that they are older (61 percent), admit they are more outspoken than they were in the past (68 percent), and say they are making an effort to do what they have always dreamed of doing (57 percent).

Three major conclusions from the report showed that:

- Age is no longer a useful indicator of how older women are living.
- Many like to see older faces in brand communications as long as those depictions are honest and authentic.
- Stereotypes are outdated. The time has come to unite, not divide the generations.

Additionally, these women felt that style should not be defined by age. They do not want to be invisible, and they wish—as if we didn't know this—for clothes that fit, flatter, and make us feel confident.

It's a firm stand on how we see ourselves. I have always felt that Frenchwomen have never looked at clothes, generally speaking, as "age-appropriate." Rather, they ask, "Does what I'm wearing make me look and feel chic?" Frenchwomen in their sixties wear tennis shoes with long summer skirts, off-the-shoulder blouses, skirts above their knees, and T-shirts beneath a tuxedo jacket. If they have great arms, they show them. And, most interesting, they don't see these ways of choosing their clothes as breaking rules. They wear what makes them feel *bien dans leur peau* (good in their skin). It's the irresistible combination of style and attitude.

As Mathilde says, "Never think it's all about the clothes. It's also the attitude we bring to what and how we wear them." Indeed.

While Mathilde is seriously submerged in the business of fashion, she believes that her position gives her a lucid insight into style. "I don't think we should work too much on ourselves or become obsessed with clothes," she says. "I do love clothes and I do love to dress up, but it's not an obsession. I like to watch what each season is offering and then choose carefully. I choose from the heart, and then I think about what I already own. Clothes should adapt to circumstances. I like to dress for occasions. It's so much fun."

She continues, "As we age, I think we should reconsider the style and color of our hair—maybe we need a change. I also think we shouldn't be too tan or too skinny, and perhaps it might be a good idea to retire stilettos. If we're not comfortable in our clothes, we're not elegant and the allure disappears."

Mathilde finds perfection in the straightforward combination of a sweater and a skirt. The pairing makes for a flawless fashion foundation. Imagine the possibilities.

When I asked the indisputable, one-of-a-kind Inès de la Fressange, who recently entered her sixth decade, what advice she would offer about cultivating one's style after a certain age, she offered these observations:

- ❀ "Wear less jewelry together."
- ❀ "Do not add too many accessories."
- ❀ "Go into the juniors' or boys' departments to buy T-shirts and wear them instead of a silk blouse under a jacket."
- ❀ "Forget about glittery makeup."
- ❀ "Instead of criticizing, be open to new things, from clothes to experiences."
- ❀ "Do not try to look twenty."
- ❀ "Smile." (She always smiles.)

STYLE IS A CONSTANT

As I've said before, one of the greatest compliments a Frenchwoman can receive is, "I love you in that dress." She doesn't care that her friends or coworkers have seen her in the same dress or suit or jacket on many occasions. She looks and feels comfortable, confident, and chic, and it shows. (It's more than likely that she changes her accessories with each wearing.)

"Maybe this is the thing," Inès suggests. "Give the impression that you have a particular style, but slightly adopt new trends. Many women keep the style they had when they were thirty. I think it's good to be aware of what's going on and evolve in a different way; this does not oblige one to become a fashion victim."

Camille Miceli, jewelry designer for Louis Vuitton, is one of Mathilde's BFFs. Mathilde gave me her cell phone number, adding, "Tell her I said she *must* meet with you."

I wasn't surprised to discover that Camille radiates a similar stunning, ebullient charm as Mathilde. It makes sense that they are such good friends. Camille perfectly describes what she brings to her style as "insouciance and spontaneity."

On the morning we met in Paris, she wore no makeup, her hair was slicked back and twisted into a tight, low chignon, and she was wearing a black dress that could have taken her from our morning coffee to a black-tie dinner, including her sky-high sandals. She looked marvelous.

She says she dresses for her mood each day, and sometimes if the weather is a little dreary and she is not feeling particularly sunny, she will turn to her closet for a happy solution. "Style is innate," she says. "It mirrors our personality, reflects a mood, transmits an esprit. We all have our insecurities, but we must set them aside—forget about them—and accept who we are and how we are. It's essential. We have to decide to feel good about ourselves."

I asked everyone I interviewed for this chapter to talk about a few of her favorite things, those clothes and accessories that unfailingly deliver chic, comfort, and confidence.

"Let me just say, I do not believe *aux tendances* [in trends]," Camille proclaims up front. "For me, every woman should appropriate *la mode* in her own way." In her own way, then, here are some of Camille's favorite things:

1) *A black knit A-line Azzedine Alaïa dress, slightly above the knee*

2) A white Louis Vuitton zippered top with little studs

3) A gray chimney-collar T-shirt

*4) A flowered Givenchy dress from the spring 2008
collection.*

5) A black leather bolero from the 1980s

*6) A tweed jacket that was her son's when he was ten
years old*

*7) A Gilles Dufour crewneck cashmere sweater (He is
Mathilde's uncle.)*

8) A black felt Commes des Garçons coat

*9) A long, gray jersey Louis Vuitton dress from the
spring 2017 collection, which she wears with
ballerina flats during the day and stilettos at night*

*10) A collection of John Smedley jerseys in black, beige,
and navy*

Camille often cuts her American Apparel T-shirts to give
them rough boat necklines. She also likes to wear brooches
with her T-shirts. "I do wear pants, but generally dresses are
easier for me—slip one on and go," she says. "And remember,"
she cautions in the middle of her clothes list, "elegance is a
way of being, it's one's comportment. Without respect and
good manners toward others, it makes no difference what
you're wearing."

As I mentioned in a previous chapter, I am a huge fan of
the elegant Christine Lagarde, the first female managing
director of the International Monetary Fund. For years I
have longed to meet her, and I finally did, though briefly, at
a party in Bordeaux. She could barely walk into the soirée

because she has lots of fans, but she kindly agreed to speak with me for a few minutes after dinner.

If you are familiar with the way she dresses, you can see that she has great style, never once thinking that she should wear uptight suit uniforms to look more businesslike, buttoned up, or masculine. She does wear trousers on occasion, but she mostly opts for dresses and skirts with matching or unmatched jackets. She dons knee-high boots, mostly medium-height heels, and evening gowns that expose just enough skin. She is utterly feminine without a soupçon of froufrou. She is the ultimate example of dressing for success. Breaking constricting rules are some of her best style lessons for all of us.

"Women do not need to dress like men," she says. Her best advice for women in business or a predominantly male profession? "Don't show too much, and always be yourself."

THE ESSENTIALS

If you read my last book or visit my blog, you have met my friend Babette Fournier. She owns several boutiques, two of which—one selling clothes, Côté Rue, and the other, À Mi Chemin, accessories and shoes—are in the town where we do our shopping. I do quite a lot of shopping chez Babette, particularly for my daughter. I love her taste and the way she buys the clothes for her shops.

One of my favorite exercises with her is to have her choose a single item from a season and then style it for three generations of women: a grandmother, *la grand-mère,* age sixtysomething; a mother, *la merè*, age fortysomething; and a daughter, *la fille* (*la petite fille* for her grandmother) age eighteen. Babette's customers range in age from fourteen to eightysomething, which in itself is proof that she knows how to assemble collections. "I buy for my boutiques the way I think is most intelligent for women to shop for themselves, which is to say eighty to eighty-five percent 'basics' and the rest fashion trends," she says.

A "basic" for Babette can be a navy blazer, but it might be piped in gold braid. A blue and white–striped poplin shirt I bought for Andrea could be considered basic and could be worn for years. The shirt is collarless, with buttons down the back and a slight peplum. It's also long enough to be tucked in if you're not in a peplum sort of mood.

Babette did two collections for a family. For the first outfit, she chose a sweatshirt top, pronounced by her as a "sweet" shirt, upon which she wanted to build the three outfits.

"No, you can't do that," I say. "We Americans have an unhealthy relationship with that garment. Many women think of sweat suits—the top and bottom separated or together—as street wear. Please choose something else." I then launched into my standard conversation about how we both knew that sweats are to be worn only in a gym and that Frenchwomen wouldn't dream of wearing them on the street. And even when they wear them in a gym, there is nothing sloppy about the fit.

STILL, SHE PERSISTED: "You don't understand," she says. "I'm talking about a 'shape,' not a literal sweatshirt, and they come in many different materials. I don't buy big, shapeless versions. I consider them a wardrobe basic, just large enough to be comfortable and not too bulky to be belted." OK, then, I acquiesced.

This is how she styled a gray sweatshirt for our intergenerational family from either Essential Apparel or Isabel Marant, depending upon the season, as those are her two favorite sweatshirt labels:

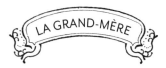

- Sweatshirt, cuffs turned back
- Lots of white pearls
- Navy straight-leg wool, linen, or Spandex-blend trousers
- Straight, pale gray, three-quarter wool coat
- Repetto patent-leather moccasins

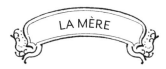

- Sweatshirt
- Bottle-green cotton sateen knee-length pencil skirt
- Black wool blazer
- Black opaque tights
- Black leather heels—"not too sophisticated, not too pointed, not too round-toed"
- Large gold cuff bracelet
- Very large brooch with lots of colored stones, including green

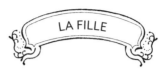

LA FILLE

- Sweatshirt tucked carelessly into the front of the pants
- "Carrot" trousers in a wool-linen blend in a gray Prince de Galles plaid, with cuffs turned up slightly
- White Converse high-tops
- A black Perfecto jacket
- Her mother's or grandmother's Hermès scarf folded into a triangle, then folded over several times into a band and tied twice around the neck
- Lots of rings

The second item for our family's outfit base was a crisp white cotton long-sleeve collarless shirt, hitting mid–hip bone (that way, it can be worn in or out):

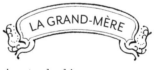

LA GRAND-MÈRE

- The chemise, tucked in
- Dark blue straight-leg Lee jeans
- A multicolored silk scarf at the neck
- Multicolored sandals in the summer
- Very feminine derby shoes in navy and silver
- Colorful socks to add interest to the shoes
- Silver *creole* (hoop) earrings
- A French-blue three-quarter coat

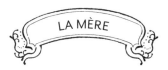

LA MÈRE

- Chemise worn unbuttoned to expose the slightest hint of décolletage
- Charcoal-gray "carrot" trousers in a wool-linen blend with the shirt tucked in
- Waist accented with a wide black-leather obi belt
- Anniel panther ballerina flats
- A gray pinstriped coat
- Gold *creole* (hoop) earrings and a mass of gold bangles on one wrist
- A yellow leather chain-link shoulder bag

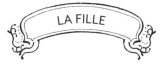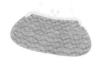

LA FILLE

- The chemise, tucked in
- A mid-thigh navy wool miniskirt with four navy buttons on each of the front sides
- Navy or black opaque tights
- Flat black lace-up *bottines*
- A ribbed navy watch cap
- A beige trench coat
- A large "washable" tattoo on one hand (so as not to make her mother and grandmother hyperventilate)

On another register, I asked Chanel's director of communications, Marie-Louise de Clermont-Tonnerre, whom I have known for decades, to tell me what she would include in a pared down twenty-piece wardrobe. "That's way too much," she says, chiding me. Like others in the business of haute fashion, Marie-Louise has access to some of the most magnificent clothes in the world, yet she maintained that it doesn't take a bursting closet to be stylish and elegant.

Like Mathilde, Camille, and Inès, she emphasizes the rule that all women with style know instinctively: "Never, ever dress from head to toe in a 'total' look. The personality comes into dressing with the way a woman makes her signature mélange."

Marie-Louise, a woman of a certain age as she happily recounts, takes very good care of herself, but then she'll say quite frankly: "*Merci Maman, merci Papa*," referring to her good luck in the gene pool. She was at Chanel before Karl Lagerfeld arrived and has been at his side ever since. She explains that he took the supremely ladylike grande-dame look that was the image of La Maison Chanel in the 1980s and added a "*coup de jeunesse*" (a shot of youth), a youth that women of every age understood.

Nevertheless, among Marie-Louise's abbreviated wardrobe, she offers sage counsel for women of a certain age. THIS IS WHAT SHE TELLS ME:

- "We live in a world that involves *la mode*, so we must evolve and make an effort. It keeps us feeling good about ourselves."
- "Less makeup."
- "Take good care of our hair; hair should always be fun, no matter how old we are."
- "After a certain age, very long hair is not flattering.

It looks like you're trying too hard."

❧ "The attitude, not the clothes themselves, is the greatest luxury we bring to dressing."

❧ "When you're finished dressing, the overall impression should be *decontracté*." (This means easy or relaxed—that famous French notion that you spent absolutely no time thinking about what and how you were going to wear your ensemble.)

❧ "One of the worst errors for a Frenchwoman is to be overdressed."

❧ "Be extremely vigilant about proportion—lengths of jackets, skirts—and make certain you are working with the most flattering cuts."

❧ "For most women over sixty, I think they might need to cover their arms—at least partially."

❧ "No bare cleavage, please."

❧ "No lip injections, *s'il vous plaît!*"

❧ "If a woman has pretty legs, she should show them. That does not mean she needs to expose her thighs."

❧ "What was elegant at thirty might not be elegant at sixty."

Marie-Louise went on to emphasize that style and elegance have "nothing to do with price. It's a way of living," she says. As for her minimal wardrobe, this is what she would want in her closet:

1) Two pairs of well-cut trousers for weekends

2) One pencil skirt for work

3) A cashmere twinset—"You can do so much with a

> *cardigan and a crewneck sweater."*
> *4) A tweed suit with matching skirt and pants and the jacket nipped at the waist*
> *5) A mousseline blouse that dresses up everything: trousers and long and short skirts*
> *6) A trench coat*
> *7) A blue blazer with blue tweed lapels*
> *8) A close-to-the-body black velvet jacket*
> *9) Mousseline evening pants*
> *10) Ballerina flats, mid-height heels, a good handbag, pretty gloves, and diamond earrings*

When I ask Inès what she thinks is essential in a woman's wardrobe, she offers only one item. "A navy blue sweater—it fits everyone and gives a neat and happy touch," she says.

I was hoping for more, but then she offers this advice: "The important thing is not to buy new things, but rather to be able to throw away all that is not good in our wardrobes, which is very hard," she admits, laughing.

As I was talking with all of these charming, intelligent, stylish women, I realized that among the traits they share is the *joie de vivre* they bring to their dressing style. They use their clothes to speak for them in important ways. At the same time, each one dresses in a completely different way, and perhaps that is the secret we need to accept: Style is what we make it. It truly is that *je ne sais quoi* we each bring to our wardrobes, and even if we can't always put words to the concept, we recognize it when we see it.

One imperative not to forget when examining a Frenchwoman's style is that she believes conformity is her enemy. She does not fantasize about fitting in or being a member of any particular fashion tribe. She strives to accentuate her singularity. Conformity is anathema. No matter how simple her clothes, and most do like simple garments, she will add her personal touch to the assemblage whether she's wearing jeans or a twenty-year-old LBD.

She rarely gets on the IT bandwagon, or if she does it's not born of a need to be "in" this season but because she fell for a current season's hot item by happenstance. Somehow, though, she manages to make her new bag or shoes or jacket seem like a natural fit for her style.

As with all my subjects, I ask Mathilde what she couldn't live without in her vast closet that she sheepishly admits has custom quarters for her more than 400-pair shoe collection.

The last time I saw her, at a party in Paris, she was wearing a floaty, knee-skimming black mousseline frock with vertiginous black sandals (she not only knows how to walk alluringly in the shoes, she can also run in them to catch a taxi), sparkling chandelier earrings, and a large ring perhaps imagined by her sister, Victoire de Castellane, Dior's fine-jewelry designer.

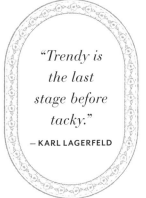

"Trendy is the last stage before tacky."

— KARL LAGERFELD

I've left her responses somewhat stream of consciousness—the way she explained them to me—but you'll see her message is clear about dressing in general:

- "If you work too much on yourself, you will no longer be natural."
- "You have to be mentally elegant in order to release an aura of style and elegance."
- "It's essential to feel comfortable in our clothes; if we're not comfortable, it shows."
- "After a certain age, we should stay away from extremes. If we like a certain color, for example, maybe it's too overwhelming after a certain point. That doesn't mean that you can't find other tones, tints, or hues of that color that are flattering."
- "Extremes also apply to skirt lengths, décolletage, makeup, and accessories."
- "Sometimes I like to dress in a coquettish way, but not by baring lots of skin. It's probably mostly attitude."
- "Pay attention to the refinement of detailing on garments."
- "Posture, posture, posture … you can't have style without good posture."
- "Less is *always* more: perfectly fitted trousers or jeans, a fitted blouse with a pullover, flat shoes, good hair, a little makeup. Simple."
- "Do make the effort to dress for occasions."

Now for her pared-down wardrobe specifics, which weren't easy for her to narrow down:

1) *A gray three-quarter Dior coat*
2) *A black-and-white houndstooth jacket to wear day and night*
3) *A shocking pink dress with its own cardigan by Azzedine Alaïa*
4) *Printed dresses from Prada*
5) *My twenty-year-old Yves Saint Laurent smoking (tuxedo) by Tom Ford. "Sometimes I'll wear it with a T-shirt, other times a blouse."*
6) *Seafarer 7 and Levi 501 jeans*
7) *All kinds of knitwear—"I love cashmere and wool."*
8) *A Little Black Dress, of course.*
9) *Lots of wool leggings*
10) *Lots of pashminas and scarves*
11) *Evening bags*
12) *All sorts of shoes and boots*

Mathilde confesses that she has a difficult time separating from her clothes and accessories. "I really love a lot of what I own," she says, "and many remind me of special moments, so it's extremely hard to say goodbye."

From Idea to Reality

Please don't think that the observations and counsel from these chic women immersed in the fashion world are too complicated or abstract or expensive. They are none of that. Trust me.

When Mathilde talks about flowered Prada dresses, think, Ah, maybe I could find a flowered dress, perhaps in a vintage boutique. That might be a pretty change. Or how about a black-and-white tweed herringbone or houndstooth jacket, possibly from the men's or boys' departments—both less expensive than in the women's department. Then if the fit is slightly off, take the new jacket to a tailor. Maybe you'll want it to be slightly closer to the body. The most important detail is that the shoulders fit—if not, don't buy the jacket.

When Camille says she loves large brooches on her T-shirts, steal the idea. When Babette builds a three-generational outfit from a collarless white shirt, see if you can find one. I intend to do just that. I don't own a collarless shirt, and when she started talking about it, all I could think about was wearing it under a V-neck sweater, cuffs turned back to show the shirt, with necklaces and scarves. Now I'm thinking of the men's department, the same place where I found a divine pleated-front, wing-collared tuxedo shirt about fifteen years ago.

When Marie-Louise explained the beauty of a mousseline blouse, see if you can find one that fits into your lifestyle. Or try the black velvet blazer-like jacket she mentioned, with detailing on the lapels. It's all good advice for the taking.

When Inès suggested a navy blue crewneck sweater as a "happy" addition to any wardrobe, remember her words when shopping. (I already have two: one large and long, the other waist-length and closer to the body. I wear them all the time.)

My point is that ideas are everywhere, and even though these women have practically unlimited access to some of the most beautiful garments in the world, each one, in her own inimitable way, is the catalyst that makes the clothes come alive. Be your own catalyst.

Many, many years ago, I interviewed the gentle and delightful director of the Musée des Arts Décoratifs for a magazine article I was writing about *l'art de vivre à la française*. I arrived with my list of questions and, as always in a good interview, the conversation zigzagged onto other subjects. I will never forget one of the most fascinating stories he told me about appreciating beauty and elegance.

I'm paraphrasing, but the gist of what he said was that exposure to the beautiful trains the eye and the intellect to recognize it. His reference was to the relationship between the kings and the court of France with the burgeoning bourgeoisie class of artisans and artists and the magnificent results of their collaborations.

He maintained that we could learn to be discerning and appreciative connoisseurs of lovely things and advocate for active rather than passive observation. "Go to museums, learn about color, look at the intricacies of fine workmanship, and teach yourself how to recognize quality," he told me at the time.

I realize it seems like I'm drifting off subject, but I'm not really. I'm using his insight to try to elucidate the abstraction of style and elegance in the subject at hand.

"Fashion is not something that exists in dresses only. Fashion is in the sky, in the street, fashion has to do with ideas, the way we live, what is happening," Coco Chanel once said.

How many times have we read or listened to interviews with designers who tell us that they find their inspiration by watching women in the street or spending hours wandering around museums? We can do the same thing. One of my favorite means of entertainment is to sit in a Parisian café and watch the world pass by. Even if some of the ideas walking down the street would never work for me, I admire the boldness or the subtle creativity and nonchalance in evidence on stylish women of all ages.

In my many years of being part of *la mode*—from the outside looking in—I discovered long ago that I do not have the personality or the audacity required to wear over-the-top fashion. At the same time, though, I love observing women who know how to play with their clothes and see the exercise as putting on a show. Why not? If they're having fun and they transmit their good humor to us, all I can think is *Merci, merci*, you brought a smile to my day.

A famous makeup artist told me in an interview for my last book that Frenchwomen like an audience. "They like to be looked at and admired," he said. "They are comfortable in that role." TRANSLATION: They care what others think, they offer their viewers free entertainment, and even if they are dressing for personal reasons, they want to put their best look on display.

The Uniform

Although *uniform* may have a negative connotation, I have one and it has set me free. When I stray too far from its components, I tend to feel uncomfortable and self-conscious.

My base colors are black and navy. Within these, the components in each uniform are more or less the same: Equipment washed-silk shirts; Eric Bompard sweaters; Uniqlo

T-shirts (because their torsos and sleeves are long—such a luxury for me); tall, flat-front trousers from Lands' End; jackets from wherever I find them; coats from Chanel, Saint Laurent, Max Mara, Lands' End, and Halsbrook; satin and crepe evening trousers from the Compagnie Française de l'Orient et de la Chine in Paris; and a mousseline blouse from Chloé when Karl Lagerfeld was the label's designer. My heels have been retired. Now I only wear ballerina flats, moccasins, and sandals.

(If you come to Paris, I highly recommend a visit to the Compagnie Française, particularly if you think a pair of simple, straight pull-on satin or crepe trousers are the one thing missing from your wardrobe. They come in a plethora of colors. I own satin pairs in ruby red, Bordeaux, black, and cream and crepe ones in gray and blue. I told you I can be excessive.)

In the spring and summer, my gabardine and flannel pieces are cleaned, repaired, and stored, and the linens and cottons come out. One of my favorite outfits is an ancient Donna Karan white linen pantsuit that I wear together or as separates.

In writing this chapter, I came to the realization that my clothes purchases are usually to replace basics or add accessories, including huge scarves and ballet flats, of which I have an embarrassing number. (A few months ago, I bought a new pair in gold because I literally wore out the first pair beyond the skills of my brilliant shoe-repair man, who just rolled his eyes when he saw them.) Occasionally, I buy a new sweater or blouse, both of which I consider accessories, and if I absolutely cannot resist, yet another coat.

The Challenge

Let's say we haven't quite perfected our style or that we have decided to reexamine or refurbish our image, for whatever reason. It could be the result of a new job, retirement, an important birthday, a fluctuation in our weight, or a major change in our lives that makes us desire something new and different. Maybe we've decided it's time for some reinvention, and we want to dress for the adventure. Maybe we own way too much, and the message we would like to convey, the way we see ourselves, gets lost in the muddle.

For example, my lifestyle has dramatically changed now that 85 to 90 percent of my time is spent in the country. Most of my clothes now are what I would call "country polished," which means they can be dressed up for lunches and meetings in Paris.

So how can we approach what we have, what we need, what we do not need, and what we want? Let's call it The Challenge. I'll ask the hard questions, you'll answer, and in the end you will have clarity about what to keep and what to discard.

1) Define your lifestyle in three to five words.

_____

2) Do your clothes fit your lifestyle?

_____

3) Is your lifestyle varied, as in work, leisure, travel, and formal, or does it tend to fall primarily into one or two categories? If so, what are they?

_____

4) Do you have what you need to work and play comfortably?

_____

5) Do your clothes fit?

_____

6) If they fit, do they flatter your body?

_____

7) Do you own too many clothes?

_____

8) Describe your personality in three to five words.

_____

9) Does your wardrobe reflect your personality?

_____

10) Do you have a uniform? Does it make you feel good or as if you are in a rut?

_____

11) What kinds of clothes do you like? Have you taken the time when shopping to see what you are naturally drawn to?

_____

12) Do you need to change what you like in some way to make it better fulfill your needs and flatter your figure?

_____

13) What clothes do you wear over and over? Why?

_____

14) Do you turn to the same things in your closet because of comfort, compliments, or habit?

_____

Since my uniform is so basic in color and form, coats are the one place where I tend to be relatively fearless in my color choices. I love my thirty-five-year-old Yves Saint Laurent French blue peacoat over navy or black, particularly on a dark, dreary winter day. I'm currently thinking I would like to find a black or gray flannel pencil skirt (the ones I own don't fit, unfortunately) that I could wear with opaque tights. I'm on a mission.

Confronting the Closet

Now that we have taken The Challenge, it is time to confront the closet. The writing of this book has brought me to some serious wardrobe-reassessment decisions. No, I have no intention of changing my uniform, but I plan to purge my closets, break up with my "had a good time in you" clothes, and cull items way down to my basics. It truly is time to do just that because I wear, more or less, the same clothes every day.

If you would like to join me, this is my grand plan along with a few general observations:

1) Clearly, ruthlessly, and unequivocally gather together the clothes I wear over and over and over. They are the items that make me comfortable and confident. I will take them out in groupings of fifteen to twenty so as not to be overwhelmed.

2) Before I do anything further with my closet, I'll repeat the above with other pieces that I wear regularly and continue the mix-and-match exercise. Anything that has seen better days is out, and anything that needs alterations goes to my wonderful seamstress, Madame Sneady. The keepers go back in the closet.

3) Next out will be the clothes that fit into my overall uniform criteria, but for some reason—were they lost in the abyss?—were never worn. Why is that?

4) The above grouping will be tried on, introduced to my basic wardrobe if they pass the fit test, and then put on a three-to-six-month trial period to see if I wear them. If not, some hard decisions will have to be made.

5) The clothes I no longer wear because—I might as well be honest—they haven't fit me for years must go. This will not be easy. Maybe this is the point where I have a "get over yourself" body-image moment, wherein I admit once and forever, "You will never wear that size again; live with it."

6) My life has changed and no longer requires formal eveningwear. The Paris party invitations dried up long ago. Therefore the party dresses should go, even my beloved Valentino evening gown that hangs in a garment bag unworn for more than a decade. I have crepe, satin, and velvet trousers with appropriate tops and jackets if ever a magical invitation arrives. For dressy dinner parties with friends in the country or Paris, I'm covered.

7) The final category of clothes in my closet: the aberrations. They are the egregious errors, the ridiculous impulse buys that have been worn once or never. They do not fall into the maybe category and deserve no trial period. Out they go with a sigh of "What was I thinking?"

The Capsule Wardrobe

The key to a successful closet purge is figuring out your capsule wardrobe.So what is a capsule wardrobe? It is a collection of essential clothing items that do not go out of fashion— basically classics (or perhaps one or two spectacular pieces that are so exceptional, they almost elude definition) that include pants, skirts, coats, and jackets that stand the test of time and can be enhanced and augmented with seasonal fashion additions. A perfect capsule wardrobe consists of a well-curated closet of clothes and accessories that fit our lifestyles, our bodies, and our image of ourselves (our style) and where, ideally, everything goes with everything. The grand plan behind the theory is that less is more because we have clearly defined what best meets all of our criteria.

I suspect you knew the definition, though. For some time now, the capsule wardrobe has been the go-to formula for figuring out how to dress with style and ease with a minimum amount of clothes that reflect our vestment personalities and lifestyles. It's the translation of that discipline into the everyday that can be complicated. Believe me, I know this.

I agree that the capsule wardrobe is the most intelligent modus operandi we can apply to our wardrobes. I like the idea in pure theory, but I understand it must be flexible. We're all different, we live in places that have from one to four real seasons, and therefore our needs are not the same. Even though I have always lived in parts of the world that have four distinct seasons, my wardrobe is set up to transition seasons. I don't have a spring or winter wardrobe, per se. It's more like spring/summer and fall/winter, and then layers are added or removed.

The capsule-wardrobe hypothesis is different for all of us, I'm sure, but by definition it requires some basic, intelligent rules. It should include thirty to forty pieces per season, as in spring/summer, fall/winter clothes, not counting accessories but counting coats. In my case that works out to about 40 pieces for spring and summer and 40 for fall and winter. Maybe I'm cheating, but I don't count T-shirts and sweaters. I like to refer to that category as "accessories." However, I usually count shirts and blouses.

For the concept to work, it must be constructed upon a solid foundation of basics, including color. Frenchwomen know the secret to great style is to build on a single color family: a base of black, gray, navy, or camel sets the stage for true elegance.

Remaining on the capsule theme, wherein new items are added each season, it's not necessary to add a precise number of new pieces to what one owns. Some years you may find five irresistible items, another year perhaps ten (or one)—only you know what you need and want. I investigate with my reference materials (the aforementioned magazines and their websites), take a hard look at what needs replacing (I always hope nothing, which tends to be the case with the exception of T-shirts) and what needs repair and dry cleaning, and then ask myself if I have seen something so exciting that it would add the *je ne sais quoi* I didn't know I needed until right that second.

When I was working in a real job, usually I bought a couple of new things each season because in those days, I wanted to signal I was "on message" and really into fashion. For example, I bought a Bordeaux tweed skirted suit that I would never buy today because Bordeaux was *the* color. It's still in my closet, poor thing. It's been years since I've worn a skirt. Maybe I should try on the jacket.

We've heard the advice "If you see something you love, buy it." Perhaps, perhaps not. Experience has taught me the difference between an impulse and a good decision. I've done both. Now I apply the twenty-four- to forty-eight-hour rule. Sleep on it. If I lose sleep thinking about it, chances are I'll splurge with no regrets.

Major department stores and some boutiques have in-house professionals whose job it is to help customers find the perfect pieces to flatter their figure and enhance their style. If you're in Paris, you can make an appointment with an expert at Galeries Lafayette, Printemps, or Le Bon Marché. I've done this, and it's worth the time. They not only offer clothing ideas, but also accessories that personalize the look.

LISTS ARE MY ABSOLUTE FAVORITE THING. I always have a small Moleskine notebook in my bag with the basics of my wardrobe, one section for fall/winter and another for spring/summer. Next to each piece of clothing I will have a number, for example: black trousers, six; white linen trousers, three; black velvet jacket, one; navy blazer, two, black skirt, one; etc. When I see something I would like to buy, I can immediately flip through the pages of my notebook to see if it meets my criteria of something that will work with several items I already own. If it doesn't, is it so spectacular that I am willing to make an exception?

I cannot tell you how many times I have rebought the same things before I started to keep track of what I owned. I rationalized the rebuys as proof that I truly understood my style, which was pathetic. Now the list gives me the overview I need to be creative and budget-conscious when shopping.

Babette keeps everything she buys for her boutiques, as well as her personal wardrobe, on her phone. She applies a similar routine to see if she is missing something in her own wardrobe or for her boutiques.

Many stylish Frenchwomen have told me that they never think of dressing as preconceived outfits and claim to stand before their closets waiting for inspiration to hit. Marisa Berenson tells me she does that, adding that she doesn't understand premeditated dressing except for grand galas.

I get it, but sometimes standing in front of a closet can instill stress and uncertainty, rather than calm and ideas. For that reason, on those I-have-nothing-to-wear days, I think it's best to have an idea about a few go-to outfits. (It's not like we have to tell anyone.)

Some women like to work on their outfits with mood or inspiration boards, but I find the most creative way to invent unexpected combinations of clothes and accessories is to play around on Polyvore. As you may know, Polyvore is a "social commerce" website that allows you to create your own mood boards or "sets," which can include everything from fashion and beauty to interior decorating.

If you're not familiar with the concept, go to polyvore .com, sign up, and begin reinventing the combinations of clothes already in your closet. You'll find similar pieces so you stay on message, then choose from thousands of accessories, clothing items, and cosmetics to invent new outfits. You can also see clearly what may be missing from your closet. Many fashion sites are set up to allow you to click on items you like and send them over to your Polyvore account. In addition, you can take your own pictures either from your closet or while shopping and send them to your account. It's like paper dolls for adults.

In the end, you have clear information about what you might want to add to an existing wardrobe: a pink coat, a paisley shawl, gold shoes, a V-neck cardigan instead of a classic crewneck, the latest red nail polish hue, and so on. It's so much fun.

No-Commitment Dressing

I recently discovered a splendid way to approach dressing when I met Pascale Guasp, the founder of ElssCollection. ElssCollection is a membership or just-for-today boutique where one can rent designer clothes for special occasions, be it a glam soiree, an important business presentation, a wedding, or a "Why not?" impulse.

Pascale took her twenty years of consulting experience and opened a gorgeous eighth arrondissement boutique where women can swoop in and leave with a pricey designer frock and without plunking down thousands of Euros.

Yes, I know renting clothes is not a new concept, but the idea and the ways we can incorporate that idea into our lives has captured my imagination for the first time.

My friend Cassandra was wearing a leopard miniskirt the other day when we met for tea in Paris. She finished off the look with a black turtleneck sweater, black opaque tights, and high black boots. I tell her I think she looks adorable in her new skirt, and she confesses she is renting it for four days. "You know," she says, "it's not like it's something you would wear every day. It's one of those things everyone remembers, so I didn't want to buy it."

That's the part of the concept that appeals to me. One can rent something that is so memorable, it wouldn't fit into a wardrobe for most women who have to respect a certain budget limit. I suggest to Pascale that when she buys for her boutique, she probably concentrates on the look-at-me types of clothes a woman wouldn't necessarily buy for herself, but wants to make an impact.

"No, not at all," she says. "Frenchwomen are always discreet. Their greatest fear is to be overdressed. What a Frenchwoman wants is a dress that will take her to the office and then to a dinner or an important evening business meeting. Beautiful designer classics are very expensive. They are an important part of the seasonal collections I buy, but they have something special about them. There is always a unique detail that makes them stand out. That's why they are expensive. The materials and workmanship are beautiful," she says.

Pascale believes that renting clothes is a new form of consummation. "It's a way to buy less and yet have more," she explains. "The system corresponds to an evolution in consumerism. Women feel less encumbered, and if they fall in love with a piece they rent, they can buy it."

She found that women are often drawn to prints, but they get tired of them and therefore don't see the logic in buying them for their wardrobes. "One thing I discovered," she says, "is no one wants to wear anything yellow. I bought some pretty pieces in yellow, and they were never rented."

Her latest offering is the Empty Suitcase plan. For 99 Euros a day, visiting Paris can be a total immersion experience in not only how to eat like a Parisian, but also how to dress like one. You can arrive with the basics in a mostly empty suitcase and choose two items daily to wear wherever. Imagine dinner in a chichi restaurant clad in a designer outfit that wouldn't fit into your budget. What's more, you can take all the selfies your little heart desires and post them everywhere.

The Style Is You

I cannot stop myself from reiterating how our clothes speak volumes about who we are. As Jean Cocteau, writer, designer, artist, friend of Marcel Proust, and member of the august Académie Française, said: "Style is a simple way of saying complicated things." What an opportunity!

An intelligently chosen wardrobe—combined with just-for-us indulgences including a pedicure, manicure, pretty-without-being-froufrou underpinnings, and, *bien sûr*, perfume lets the world know that we care about ourselves. As Inès explains, "The idea is never to look wealthy, but to feel comfortable in our clothes, to seduce ourselves before seducing others." When I ask her how she would define that extra-special something so many Frenchwomen possess, she tells me, "French style is a mix of styles, vintage and new, classic and rock, ethnic and chic, casual and luxurious."

THE VERY RECIPE FOR PERSONAL STYLE is to take what we like and turn it into a singularly distinctive expression of who we are. Our capsule wardrobe, with its basic foundation (remember each of us defines *basic* differently—my blazer might be your spencer, your leather jacket might be my peacoat), hangs in our closet waiting for us to—joyfully—turn it into our sartorial story.

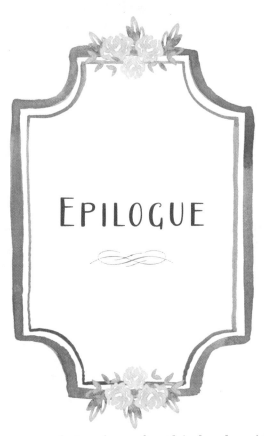

EPILOGUE

In my many interviews for this book, without exception, everyone defined *l'art de vivre* in the same way: the philosophical, historical, and daily approach to living well as a mélange of sensual, sensible, and sustaining traditions, rituals, and disciplines that bring happiness and contentment to the quotidian.

There's nothing complicated in the explanation; the execution is rather more complex, as I've discovered over the years. Paying attention to the daily details combined with the discipline it sometimes takes to stay on message is, by my definition, the secret to *l'art de vivre* and, by extension, a life well lived.

When my then-eight-year-old daughter, Andrea, and I moved to France all those years ago, we had three *very* large dogs in tow. Because of the dogs, it was impossible to live in Paris. I found a small thatched roof house west of the city with a fenced-in garden that was also home to a rather unpleasant pony as well as a divine horse. Thus began our great adventure in *l'art de vivre à la française.*

Through my vast and varied experiences over more than three decades in France, I've consciously tried to apply what I consider the best of the best from my encounters with the French people, particularly *les femmes d'un certain age,* into the way I conduct my life. I have learned more about taking the time and savoring the pleasure of purposely adhering to the rituals and routines that are the habits of my friends and acquaintances. Thanks to them, I feel my life is more productive, fulfilling, and joyful than it could have been had I not had the opportunity of being the "outsider" observing and absorbing the details of everyday life in my adopted country.

From what I admire and appreciate most about my observations and experiences with my friends and acquaintances, I've judiciously chosen the disciplines I can realistically apply to my life on a regular basis. I've taken inspiration wherever I have found it and rejected what doesn't appeal to or work for me.

When I say I've assembled my list of the best of the best from what I've learned, I'm talking about cherries in June; asparagus in March; lilacs from the garden in the spring; anemones (from the florist) in December; simple dinners and lively conversations with friends; a new wine discovery; finding yet another surprisingly delicious cheese; and cultivating relationships with the experts at our market (Laurent selects our weekly fish choices and includes recipe tips, Renaud chooses the freshest artichokes, and François tells me when it's not a good idea to buy nectarines. "Wait two weeks," he will advise). Dressing up for cocktails and dinners in Paris is good for the morale, as is savoring a tiny raspberry macaron; walking my dog in the fields behind our house in the country; gathering kindling in the Rambouillet forest for the fireplace; sharing coupes of Champagne to celebrate or commiserate; trying a new perfume; staying loyal to my classic uniform; devoting time to my beauty rituals (with major payoffs); daring to experiment with a red(!) lipstick; sitting on a terrace in Paris sipping a *chocolat chaud* watching the world go by; and attending a new exhibition followed by lunch with a girlfriend.

Andrea has transported many of her experiences to her life in Chicago, including the way she cooks, dresses, and organizes her home. (Well, she *is* a Virgo, so she probably would have organized her home even if she never set foot in France.)

Ella, my four-year-old granddaughter, eats like a French child: lots of fruits and vegetables; plain yogurt; a treat of milk, a piece of fruit, and a couple of homemade cookies after school; and no sugary treats for dessert except on special occasions, only fruit. The other day, she thought eating two M&Ms was extremely exciting. As her mother says, "We'll see how long that lasts."

L'art de vivre is most certainly an esprit, a way of looking at life as full of possibilities that make the everyday more enjoyable and, in many cases, more beautiful. Sometimes contentment is a decision waiting to be made. It makes me happy to buy a bunch of blue or white anemones in the dark days of winter, for example, or experiment with a new recipe.

I've learned so much from my French girlfriends. They have taught me that less is almost always more and that it's in our best interest to learn how to do a few things well and forget about the rest. That includes our culinary exploits, housekeeping, decorating, entertaining, and, naturally, our beauty and dressing routines. Our reputations are built upon those choices. All of them reflect our style and intentions. We are our "brand," if you think about it.

In general I find that Frenchwomen have a natural affinity for details in all aspects of their lives, and therein perhaps lies the secret to their *je ne sais quoi*. From the way they assemble an outfit to the way they set a table, the details reflect their personality. As you've seen in the previous chapters, they like organization for the simple reason that it makes everything easier. All the better if the organization is pretty and in some cases sweetly aromatic.

Sometimes I think that it's important to stress another prevalent characteristic among my friends and relations: Generally, Frenchwomen are quite frugal. They prioritize time and expenditures. They say *"non"* to protect their precious time and ask "Is it worth it?" when purchasing clothes. I'm still working on this one.

At the same time, they are extraordinarily generous in their friendships, and their loyalty is deep and abiding. They can be exceptionally charitable in excusing slights and bad behavior, far more than I.

I continue to be a work in progress on all fronts, except for the decoration of our home. That is the one area where I'm completely happy with the results. We have created a warm, charming haven in our country cottage. As for my closets, the linens are beautifully organized, but perhaps slightly overstocked; the larder needs some rethinking; we should and will be entertaining more often; and then there are my clothes, where some serious culling is necessary.

Often my husband will say to me, "You're more French than the French." And then a friend will say, "Oh, you're so American." I think that's a lovely balance, the best of the best.

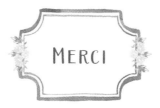

MERCI

Paris. It was love at first sight. How could it not have been?

Long before I ever thought I would live in France (where I've now been for more years than I lived in the United States), I was visiting regularly for work and play, and my affection and admiration for this wonderful country grew with each new encounter. In the back of my mind, I always thought that perhaps one day I would write a book and share what I love best about living here.

Finally, I wrote a de rigueur proposal and sent it to my supportive, hands-on, hand-holding agent and now friend, Lauren Galit, who in turn offered the idea to Rizzoli. And Rizzoli, my dream-come-true publisher, liked the idea. That was my first book, *Forever Chic: Frenchwomen's Secrets for Timeless Beauty, Style and Substance*.

But I felt, and fortuitously for me Rizzoli agreed, that there was so much more to say about living forever chic. I wanted to explore the world of *l'art de vivre à la française* in depth, and this new book is the result.

My experiences and observations have taught me that applying the notion of *l'art de vivre* to every detail in life is an exquisite way to make each day more agreeable. I decided I could have all the opinions in the world on the subject, but no one knows more than those who have been enthusiastically embracing the philosophy since childhood.

In the scores of interviews I conducted for the book, I met the kindest, funniest, most generous, and most interesting people.

One of the happiest moments was when I reconnected with Françoise Dumas, who I had not seen for two decades and who knows absolutely *everyone* and their cell phone numbers. We sat down with tea and chocolates in her Paris office as she went through the list of her friends she thought I must contact. "Just say I suggested you call them," she said. I did, and without exception all of her recommendations are in the chapters.

One of my favorite people *ever* is Kathleen Jayes, my editor at Rizzoli. Her delicate, intelligent, crisp editing made this book, like the one before, infinitely better. I am eternally grateful to her and consider myself lucky that we have become friends over the years.

I cannot begin to express my appreciation for the affection and support I have received from those who have followed and encouraged me on my blog. If I could name every one, I would.

A short list of friends, old and new, who mean the world to me: Judy, Betty Lou, Sharon, Marsi, Lesley, Mary Carol, Annette (both of you), Susan, Cassandra, and my adorable son-in-law, Will Fletcher, who is a constant cheerleader.

Merci mille fois to you for reading my book. I hope you have had as much enjoyment reading it as I had writing it.

And of course, always and ever, nothing I do would ever be possible without the two great loves of my life, Andrea and Alexandre.

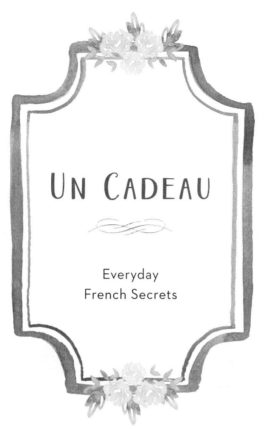

Un Cadeau

Everyday
French Secrets

In the following pages, you'll find more tips and treats you might like to try for your very own *art de vivre* à la *française*. Enjoy!

TAKING A BEAUTIFUL PHOTOGRAPH

In many French homes, Harcourt Studio portraits are part of family tradition. Some of the photographs are dramatically glamorous; others are straightforward and lovely. My husband has a collection of the widely recognizable black-and-white photographs of himself with his mother, father, and brother. For some families, these photographs are once-in-a-lifetime experiences. For others, sitting before the Harcourt camera can occur multiple times over the years. A Harcourt portrait is a rather expensive investment, which makes them precious heirlooms.

Recently I spent several hours at the Harcourt Studio— an impressive hôtel particulier in Paris's 16th arrondissement featuring one of those grand entrance staircases—interviewing its director, Catherine Renard, and sitting in on a photo session.

Catherine sees the portraits as yet another aspect of *l'art de vivre*. "We make a woman eternally beautiful," she says. "That's far better than a psychiatrist." (I thought it was far better than a plastic surgeon as well.)

"We know that our photographs become part of a family's history, and that is important for us. What we do comes from a certain perpetuation of France's royal tradition. In the past, painters captured the images of their subjects with oils on canvas. Bourgeois families wanted to be like the nobles, but with the modernity of the nineteenth century. We are part of that patrimony. Harcourt portraits transcend time. They become an immortal image that is passed down from generation to generation," she says.

I know this last part is true because every time I asked someone I know if there were Harcourt photographs on display (or tucked away) in his or her home, the answer was always yes.

The subject of the photo session I observed was Aude Extrémo, the beautiful and talented French mezzo-soprano. I sat through her makeup session, wherein the products were applied to play to the light. Harcourt photographs tend to be different from current photographic trends that focus on light-reflecting highlights. These images appear matte and more strikingly strong.

Here are a few of the tricks I learned for creating a lasting impression while being photographed:

- Before the first click of the camera, close your eyes, roll your shoulders, and breathe deeply.
- Stretch up your neck and hold your head high. This sculpts the neck and chin.
- Between shots, dip your head then raise it slowly. This prevents a tense, static expression.
- After a series of shots, stop for a moment and open your mouth wide, stick out your tongue, breathe, raise your shoulders, and release.
- Find a memory that will make you smile. "Then you will have *amour* in your eyes," Catherine says. "And it will show in the photograph."

HOMEMADE POTPOURRI

For me, even though the translation of *potpourri* means putting rotten ingredients into a pot, I am charmed by the results of the "wilted" components that smell so wonderfully romantic. Therefore, as a one-off, I decided to make my very own potpourri, just to be able to say I did it. And what follows is how I did it, if you would like to try it yourself.

1. Assemble 1 cup each of the following ingredients:

- **FLOWER PETALS AND BUDS:** roses, lavender,

violets, lilacs and lily of the valley. My suggestion is to combine at least three floral ingredients—more if you're adventurous, fewer if you want to begin slowly.

- ❧ AROMATIC LEAVES: verbena, citrus, lemon verbena, eucalyptus
- ❧ HERBS: mint and laurel leaves and rosemary
- ❧ SPICES: cloves, cinnamon sticks, and those pretty pinky-red peppercorns for color
- ❧ CITRUS (OPTIONAL): Depending upon my mood, I'll use thinly cut strips of grapefruit, orange, lemon, lime, clementines, and bergamot, or combinations thereof.
- ❧ ESSENTIAL OILS: I like the freshness of citrusy oils, but you might prefer herbal, floral (such as the classic lavender), or spicy oil, and, of course, you can mix them. Start slowly with four or five drops. Mix gently, so as not to break the petals and leaves. Begin with a drop or two of the oils you like best to arrive at the combinations you like best. You are the perfume "nose" of your creation.

2. Dry the ingredients: For the herbs and flowers, you may do this in a traditional oven on a parchment-covered cookie sheet for at least two hours at 200°F (approximately 95°C), or in a microwave. The petals and leaves should be crisp to the touch; if not, continue "baking" in 10-minute intervals until they are.

For the microwave (my method), place the flower petals, leaves, and buds on a large plate covered with a paper towel. Heat on high for two minutes and check to see if the petals "crack" to the touch. If not, heat again in 30-second intervals.

The system for the citrus is slightly more complicated: Place the pieces on a cookie sheet, and bake in a 280°F (140°C) oven for one hour with the door of the oven slightly open. Let cool.

3. Gently mix the cooled ingredients together in a glass bowl with the spices and let it rest. I let my mixture "sleep" until the next day. I've also found that when I have had stimulation overdose with all the ingredients, it's best that I, too, rest to better judge the fragrance the next day. If you want a stronger scent, a few drops of essential oil can be added.

NOTE: To "fix" or stabilize the perfume of the potpourri, some French recipes recommend adding chopped orris (iris) root. After extensive research, I discovered the measure is about four heaping tablespoons. Orris root also contributes a lovely fragrant violet note to the composition.

Since the fragrance will gradually dissipate, the potpourri can be refreshed with a spray of essential oil (or oils) concocted with 20 drops of oil to one tablespoon of water. Gently mix with your hands by letting the potpourri slip through your fingers.

LES JOIES DU VIN

Since wine is such an integral part of *l'art de vivre* and, by extension, joie de vivre, I couldn't resist sharing some of the vocabulary, definitions, and fun facts I learned while

A VINIFICATION VOCABULARY

Alcool: the alcohol in the composition derived from the fermentation process when yeast cells convert the sugar from the grape juice into alcohol; it's the alcohol that gives a wine its "warmth"

Ampélographie: the scientific field concerned with the identification and classification of *cépages* (grapevines)

A.O.C.: the *Appellation d'Origine Contrôlée* (Appellation of Controlled Origin), delineating the geographic limit from where a wine may originate and by what methods it may be made, specifically regulated under French law

Appellation: the geographic origin of a wine's grapes

Blanc de Blancs: "white from white"—white wines made from only white grapes—primarily used in Champagne, which is made from Chardonnay grapes

Cépage: the grape variety

Cru Classé: the rankings or classifications of the great wines from Bordeaux châteaux

Élevage: a wine's "maturation" or "raising" as the process moves between fermentation and bottling

Fermentation: the transformation of the grapes' sugar into alcohol when it interacts with yeast

Fût: the oak barrel used in a wine's aging process

Millésime: the year the grapes were harvested to produce the wine; the vintage

Mousseux: effervescence

Moût: the juice of the pressed grapes before the fermentation process

Oenologie: the science of wine making

Oenophile: a person who loves and perhaps studies wine

Raisin de Cuve: the grapes destined to make wine

Raisin de Table: the grapes we eat at the table

Terroir: the combination of the soil, climate, variety of grapes, and *savoir faire* of the winemaker

Vendanges: the grape harvest

Vin de Cépage: a wine made from a single grape varietal, such as Chardonnay, Cabernet Sauvignon, Pinot Noir, Riesling, or Merlot

Vinification: the transformation of grape juice into wine by fermentation

Vin Nouveau: the first wine of a vintage, meant to be consumed immediately; Beaujolais Nouveau, for example, may be available within weeks of the *vendanges*

A DÉGUSTATION VOCABULARY

Ample: a harmonious wine that gives the sensation of filling the mouth while leaving a pleasant, lasting taste

Boisé: oaky aromas (*boisé* means "woody") that develop during the wine's aging process in wood barrels; one can identify traces of coffee, chocolate, or vanilla

Bouquet: the mature aromas that develop with age in fine wines

Chaleureux: a wine that, by its alcohol content, gives the impression of warmth in the mouth

Corpulent: a robust, full-flavored red wine

Décantation: transferring wine from its bottle into a carafe in order to separate its *dépôts*, or sediments, while at the same time aerating it and releasing its aromas

Effervescent: wines with bubbles of gas

Elégant: a well-balanced wine without being overly aggressive or strong

Epicé: "spicy" aromas like pepper or tobacco, which can be the result of barrel aging or the characteristics of specific grapes used to make the wine

Equilibre: a well-balanced wine featuring a pleasant harmony between the fruit, alcohol, acidity, and tannins

Féminin: a wine said to express finesse and elegance

Fin: a pleasant, light-bodied wine that is subtle, delicate, and "softer" on the palate

Finale: the final impression on the palate, a wine's "finish"; the longer the flavor lingers, the more sophisticated the wine

Harmonieux: a wine in balance and harmony with all of its ingredients

Intense: a concentrated wine with a rich bouquet and vibrant color

Larmes: the oily traces (literally "tears") running down a glass after the wine is swirled, which gives an idea of its viscosity and some indication of its levels of alcohol, sugar, and glycerin

Longueur: a wine that leaves a lingering flavor in the mouth, usually signifying high quality

Moelleux: a sweet, "soft" wine

Opulent: a rich, well-constructed wine

Parfumé: the floral sensation given by some aromatic wines

Puissant: strong, full-flavored wines with a rich bouquet and often high levels of alcohol

Riche: a deep, full-bodied, complex wine

Rond: a smooth, well-balanced wine that gives the impression of "rolling" on the tongue

Sage: a "correct," harmonious wine without pretention or intensity

Suave: a pleasant, well-balanced, harmonious wine

Vert: a "green," young wine that has not aged sufficiently

Viril: a wine that is robust, strong, and full-flavored

writing this book. More than that, I think of these offerings as marvelous opportunities for conversation. And, as we all know, vibrant conversation—even better when enjoyed with wine—is one of the most pleasurable pastimes in a life well lived.

CASHMERE CARE

I am absolutely mad about cashmere and have an embarrassing number of crewneck pullovers, cardigans, V-necks, and turtlenecks (not to mention my oversized cashmere scarves, which I use to change my daily uniform into something more fashion-y and fun). Just recently, I bought a black cashmere "blazer" with zipper details.

I also recently had the pleasure to interview Eric Bompard, owner and visionary behind the eponymous French luxury cashmere line. I asked him how to best handle my bounty with the care it deserves. His tips are simple, but essential to keep cashmere in beautiful condition for many years.

"Cashmere loves water and should be washed often," Eric Bompard tells me. "Sweaters should be washed after two, maximum three, wearings. I think 'serious' luxury cashmere enters into a woman's life around the age of twenty, and from that first experience, there is no turning back."

Except for those with sophisticated adornments, sweaters can be washed in a machine, preferably in a lingerie bag on a cold-water cycle combined with a few drops of product (back to this in a second), with a slow rinse-and-tumble cycle. Think delicates when washing cashmere. *Never* add fabric softeners to the wash.

We all know the drill for drying: flat on a purpose-made sweater rack or a towel, carefully reshaped to its original form and kept away from sunlight.

Remember, if you prefer handwashing, don't twist or wring the garment. Soak, gently squeeze out the water, and lay flat.

Pretreat spots before washing with a tiny dab of K2r, and remove any pilling with a special sweater comb. According to Eric Bompard, pilling has nothing to do with the price of cashmere. "Even the most expensive sweaters will have some pilling, and with regular washings, you'll notice there will be much less," he says. Fine cashmere voile scarves and shawls should be dry-cleaned.

I wanted more information, so I turned to my wonderful Australian friend, who is editorial director of *Vogue Knitting* magazine, the divine Trisha Malcolm. When I ask her what she thinks about all the chatter that claims we can wash cashmere using baby shampoo, she is typically direct: "I wouldn't," she says.

Instead, she says that the absolute best product is Eucalan, which she explains is totally natural and has lanolin that functions as a "conditioner" for delicate cashmere fibers.

"I grew up with it and have been using it my entire life," Trisha says. "It is pH neutral and available either unscented or in five essential-oil fragrances. You need only a small amount and very little water, and you don't have to rinse the product out—it is biodegradable and gives some protection against moths. You can, of course, put your sweaters in a lingerie bag in the machine, but I prefer handwashing because the less agitation, the longer sweaters will last."

Now for protecting our precious purchases. Both Trisha and Eric Bompard emphasize—several times—that we must never store our sweaters unless they are pristine and clean, otherwise we are preparing nice, cozy, delicious homes for moths.

After washing sweaters and dry-cleaning scarves, thoroughly clean closet shelves and drawers before returning garments to their homes, then add an appropriate moth-deterring element like balls of cedar, which Eric recommends and which can be refreshed by adding more cedar oil.

Bompard sweaters come with linen bags, which I use to store my clean cashmere and wool items.

Trisha also suggests a solution, totally unbeknownst to me, to killing moths or larvae if they live *chez nous*: freezing. "To kill moths and moth eggs, put the clean, wet garment in a plastic freezer bag and place in the freezer for at least seventy-two hours. Remove and lay flat to defrost and dry," she says.

SEASONAL BOUQUETS WITH CATHERINE MULLER

It was the first day of spring when Catherine Muller, floral designer and teacher extraordinaire (see page 56 for more on her flower school), and I had our final interview. As I look out at our garden from the kitchen window, I lament that the barely there forsythia blossoms were dusted with snow.

"Oh, oh," Catherine says. "No, don't worry, it will probably be OK." (She was right.)

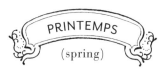

We have a conversation about seasonal bouquets, and I ask her to describe one each for spring, summer, fall, and winter, plus something small and pretty for a *Noël* dinner table (or for any end-of-year holiday).

It's not at all surprising that Catherine is passionate about her profession, but more than her love of flowers and the decorative elements in creating beautiful bouquets, she is enchanted by nature, so much so that she loves to pluck wheat from fields, wildflowers from forests, and branches from trees and bushes in gardens. In her poetic approach to the subject, here is how Catherine envisions each season:

PRINTEMPS
(spring)

"When you look at a garden in the spring, you'll see the branches and leaves are reaching toward the light. The feeling is definitely rebirth, vitality, lots of expression. In the beginning nothing is quite open, but rather 'arriving,' and I want to convey that impression in a bouquet.

"I like to use branches of cherry blossoms, parrot tulips, Christmas roses, wild hyacinth, freesias, grape hyacinth, and deep Bordeaux hellebores. This bouquet is a celebration of a garden's bounty after a long winter, and therefore it is colorful and gay. It's a mélange of pale pink, light and dark oranges, and wine hues, and the perfume is light, 'green' with a vegetal acidity, and fresh and invigorating.

"This would be a large, high arrangement, and I would put it in a transparent vase where you could see the stems and branches in the water. I would leave some blossoms on the submerged branches, and water and the vase act as a magnifying glass.

"It's important to remember that tulips prefer that you 'forget' them, which means leave one or two inches of water in the vase and don't worry about everyday water changes. The less water given to bulb plants, the happier they are."

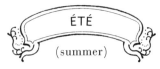

ÉTÉ
(summer)

"I take my inspiration from fields of grain and tall, wild grasses this time of the year. I love the way the stalks bend in a light summer breeze and reach out for the warmth of the sun. This is the moment when the roses are lush and fully open—they expose their hearts for us.

"Again, this is a tall, imposing bouquet with a luxurious, seductive perfume. It is composed of a mix of roses, all in pale blush tones, with a few wild roses for their simplicity next to the more sophisticated blooms (my favorites are Prince Jardinier, Fox Trot, Iceberg, O'Hara, and Pierre de Ronsard); branches of blackberries; stems of mint and lemon-scented geranium leaves, to add a more complex structure to the perfume; and stalks of grasses like *Panicum virgatum* (switchgrass) and *Pennisetum* (fountain grass).

"I would put this bouquet, which is about three feet tall, in an old grayish-beige terra-cotta pot and let all the elements arrange themselves. What you want is a mix of the sophisticated with the humble, so you let nature do the arranging. Remember, the vessel should not be more important than the flowers it holds. The perfume with the mingling of the seductive rose scents and the mint and lemon is magical."

A NOTE ABOUT ROSES: "They are capricious and like lots of attention, therefore their water should be changed every day and a tiny bit of the stem should be cut off."

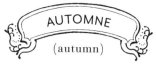

AUTOMNE
(autumn)

"With the shorter days, the garden can feel a little melancholic. The pigmentation on the flowers in bloom has changed. Still, it is a time that provides interesting ideas for bouquets. I like to collect graduated shades of mustard, amber, and wine. I also think of 'collecting' rather than arranging, which is to say I put together what I choose in the crook of my arm in a nonchalant way without structure.

"In autumn, I like to mix chestnut branches, white *symphorine* berries, branches of oak leaves, amaranth foxtail, dahlias, hydrangeas, heather, and bishop's-weed.

"I have a collection of old, rustic baskets that I've found over the years at flea markets that I would use for this arrangement. I put a plastic container with the water inside the basket."

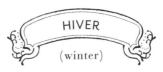

HIVER
(winter)

"The gardens are resting now, and the only 'courageous' flowers one might see are snowdrops and cyclamen. In the winter, my concentration is directed toward the vast variety of resinous trees. There are so many varieties and nuances of colors, from bright greens to blue and gray greens.

"I tend to like making wreaths, but not with a very structured form. I let the branches dictate the shape. I try to find one large pliable branch that I can easily bend to form the base, then build on it with different types of pine variations and colors. If 'woven' together, the pieces will support the whole, but it's also possible to use floral wire to keep everything in place. Then I add small pine cones and bluish or white berries. If you like the contrast, holly berries can be lovely.

"Let's say, though, that one might prefer not to try the wreath challenge. It is possible to make a gorgeous winter or holiday bouquet from the branches decorated with berries. Because the berries dry more quickly than the boughs and tend to fall off, it's a good idea to affix them with floral glue. The branches should last one to two months. (Keep the branches in a small amount of water for one week, then remove water for the duration.) The fragrance of the mélange of pine will fill the house and lift the spirits.

"I imagine the boughs in a large, unpolished silver or bronze urn, not something too shiny."

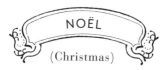

NOËL

(Christmas)

"For a holiday table at this time of year, it would be pretty to see a collection of burnished silver *timbales* (silver tumblers) with white anemones, a few sprigs of pine or mistletoe, and tiny Christmas balls in white or silver."

Her ideas are lovely, non?

In the winter, when I can't pop out the door to gather a bouquet from the garden and I haven't been to the florist—or the grocery store—I cut branches of crimson leaves from my Red Robin bushes and mix them with the hydrangea blooms I dry every year and the lavender I harvest from the garden in the fall. I've had great success with my hydrangea and lavender. Both last through the winter. (It's now possible to buy reasonably priced flowers at many grocery stores, whereas a few years ago, the concept had not caught on in France.)

We also have a bounty of pine cones because our garden is full of pine trees. They're perfect for building a fire in the fireplace, or you can spray them gold or silver for the holidays to fill a silver Revere bowl. They are instant decoration.

I refuse to use artificial flowers. I realize some women will disagree with me, but I find the idea of flowers that need to be dusted quite off-putting. These days, at least at our nursery, there are many varieties of moderately priced orchid plants. I have at least one, usually two, in the salon and another on my desk, and I have managed to keep them alive for several months. They are my alternative to *faux fleurs*, they last and last, and they are real.

SECRETS OF *LE RÉGIME FRANÇAIS*

Until I met renowned chef Michel Guérard, I was convinced that there was nothing more to be said about dieting. How wrong I was. He has proven that it's possible to create spectacularly delicious, healthy, low-calorie French recipes.

"Taste and enjoyment lie at the heart of all French cooking," Michel Guérard says, "so I'm drawn to conclude that any plan to reform eating habits must not lose sight of the fact that people want to enjoy their food. Any sort of cooking or diet is doomed to failure if it fails to give pleasure.

"For the French, eating is one of the most instant and accessible routes to pleasure. It is a pleasure to which we feel entitled as human beings. You might even say that we regard it as an inalienable social right. But the French do not want to choose between health and pleasure; they want both at the same time."

Eating well is a French obsession, and Michel Guérard revels in the challenges and discoveries involved in concocting exciting new culinary masterpieces. "In order to succeed, any healthy-eating regime must be rooted in social custom, which means that its meals must include an element of ritual and special moments of enjoyment, whether or not they are shared with others," he adds.

"It's counterproductive when a regime is a form of punishment. I wanted to develop a *cuisine minceur* [slimming cuisine] that was satisfying and pleasurable." Mission accomplished.

Based on Michel Guérard's rigorous culinary research and experimentation, Minceur Essentielle was born in 1975.

The program was created for those who wished to lose weight without sacrificing pleasure, all against the backdrop and thermal-water treatments of the Guérards' breathtakingly beautiful Les Prés d'Eugénie hotel and spa. He refers to his method as losing weight "serenely," and indeed it is.

I spent an "all-in" intensive one-week immersion program at the spa. My *régime* program included consultations with the director of the thermal-water spa, Cécile Ledru, who is also an aesthetician using the luxe Sisley cosmetic line on offer in the spa (more on that on page 153–154); Cécile Guionnet, the dietitian who not only weighed and measured me, but also calculated my muscle mass, body water, and fat; and fitness coach Grégory Bats, whose name I momentarily forgot because I was trotting so quickly on the treadmill, I was in a panic and didn't take notes.

While many diners were consuming delightful inventions from the "real" menu, those of us on the slim *régime* were given our menus, with the chef's choices of each day's lunch and dinner featuring the meals' calorie counts beneath their respective desserts. We were always asked if we were pleased with what was on offer. One would be a fool not to be.

Always, always cook with the finest ingredients. That is of primary importance, Michel Guérard emphasizes. "Simplicity is an art," he says. "When cooking with the best ingredients, it's not necessary or even desirable to be complicated."

Below are some of the fundamentals on which the *cuisine minceur* pleasure principle is based. Plus, I present a few recipes I've tried with great general approval *chez nous.* There is not a moment when you think you are actually on a low-calorie diet.

1. **STOCKS AND VARIATIONS:** Michel Guérard tells us these "lie at the heart" of his approach to healthy cooking. They form the core to his vast collection of recipes and sauces, either as an integral ingredient to a dish or contributing to an accompanying sauce. He even uses them to replace or minimize the use of oil in his vinaigrettes. Ever since I arrived home, I've been using his vinaigrette recipes.

2. **FLAVORED OILS:** In his vinaigrette recipes, he calls for one quarter of the amount of oil normally used. Michel Guérard credits his friend and fellow chef, Michel Trama, for offering him technical advice in the process of making the oils.

3. **VINAIGRETTES:** These are where the stocks and flavored oils are mingled to masterful effect. I have been using low-salt bouillon cubes I buy at the grocery store, which Guérard suggests for those who do not make their own stock.

4. **CLASSIC SAUCES AND CONDIMENTS:** Long the hallmark additions to French cuisine, these have been revisited with mystifyingly delectable results.

5. **LIAISONS:** In the past, liaisons were typically based upon mixtures of flour and butter, the classic roux, or egg yolks and heavy cream—all delicious and all highly calorific. By using purees of vegetables and fruits, Michel Guérard found the perfect substitutes for thickening ingredients.

My Example
MENU

LUNCH

Entrée: *L'oeuf mollet en habit vert* (Soft boiled egg with a green vegetable sauce)

Plat: Hamburger

Dessert: *Paris-Brest au café* (hazelnut pastry)

Total Calories: 540

DINNER

Entrée: *Taboulé de jeunes legume printaniers* (Tabbouleh with young spring vegetables)

Plat: *Soufflé de noix de Saint-Jacques, sauce coraillée* (Scallop Soufflé with coral sauce)

Dessert: *Panna cotta à la verveine du jardin* (Panna cotta with garden verbena)

Total Calories: 470

6. COLD COULIS: These are emulsified sauces made from either vegetables or fruits, and based on the same principle as liaisons, which is to say they are fine purees. The cold coulis can be used as a condiment in the same way one might add mayonnaise to make a simply prepared cold meat or fish more interesting. (I've included a coulis recipe with the dessert below so you have an idea how to make a low-calorie coulis for a variety of culinary creations.)

In our interview, Michel Guérard enumerates a few important details that must be respected to succeed in the preparation of a slimming cuisine. He emphasizes the importance of exact measurements and credits the debut of his career as a pastry chef as an invaluable lesson in precision. "When making pastries, there are no approximate measurements the way there can be when preparing meals," he says.

He took his precision discipline to the creation of his slim *régime* and cautions all who wish to join him in the adventure to be equally diligent in recipe preparations. His alternatives for fats, salt, and sugar are as satisfying, or even more so, than the real thing.

Liaisons stand in for fats; salt is compensated for by using stocks (bouillon is the dehydrated version of a stock and can be used to replace a stock if you do not make your own or cannot find an equivalent in a grocery store) and marinades with taste bud–tantalizing herbs and spices. One of his favorite refined-sugar substitutes is xylitol, primarily found in the bark of the silver birch tree. (I discovered xylitol several years ago from the owner of our favorite health-food store and love everything about it.)

Good fats are used judiciously. Since they are high in calories (one tablespoon of oil is 90 calories), Michel Guérard has once again met the challenge with creativity.

Butter, let's be honest, is divine though 80 percent fat. Still, some recipes would not be the same without its irreplaceable taste. For that reason, he says "Never mind the alternatives," because they will never produce that delicious buttery taste. He has been happy with the addition of about 10 percent of the butter called for in a sauce.

He uses 2 percent milk in recipes, never zero, as fat gives flavor. Some recipes include unsweetened condensed semi-skim milk, because concentrated milk is perfect for some desserts and certain savory dishes, where it can be an ideal substitute for fats like oil or butter. (I've tried this, and it's brilliant.)

In general, his favorite cooking methods for the home include poaching, steaming, stewing, and braising in paper or foil parcels (*en papillote*), which results in rich flavors sealed into the food.

Now that we've talked about the philosophy of the essential *cuisine minceur,* let's get down to a few of his recipes, all of which I've tried. I have included in this appendix only recipes that have a one-star difficulty rating, but some recipes are two- and three-star challenges.

A FEW OF MY FAVORITE *CUISINE MINCEUR* RECIPES

These recipes are easy to make and absolutely delicious. I've included a soup as an *entrée,* two *plats* or main courses, and, *obviously,* one dessert. Then I added a little bonus, Michel Guérard's out-of-this-world recipe for *confiture* (jam).

AUTUMNAL CÈPE AND MUSHROOM SOUP

Serves 4; 75 calories per serving
Preparation time: 45 minutes

Ingredients

1 tsp. olive oil
2 oz. onions, finely sliced or chopped (I use yellow onions)
1³/₄ oz. leeks, white part only, split lengthwise and sliced into
    ¹/₂-inch pieces
6¹/₂ oz. fresh *cèpes* (porcini mushrooms), wiped and roughly chopped;
    or 3¹/₂ dried *cèpes,* soaked in water for 20 minutes, then
    squeezed and chopped, water reserved; or 6¹/₂ oz.
    frozen *cèpes*
4¹/₂ oz. white button mushrooms, wiped and quartered
Salt and pepper
1¹/₂ cups chicken stock, homemade or from a bouillon cube
1¹/₂ cups 2 percent milk
4 thinly sliced *cèpes* or mushroom of choice, grilled or roasted briefly,
    for garnish
Sprinkling of fresh, finely chopped herbs such as chervil, flat-leaf
    parsley, or chives, for garnish (optional)

Instructions

1. Heat olive oil in a saucepan over gentle heat. Add onions and leek
   and sweat them, covered, for about 2 minutes or until they have
   softened without coloring. Add *cèpes and* button mushrooms.
   Stir for about 3 minutes, or until they start to color. Season lightly
   with salt and pepper, because you will season again after reducing
   the liquid.
2. Stir in chicken stock. Bring liquid to a boil, lower heat, cover
   saucepan, and simmer gently for 30 minutes.

3. Remove saucepan from the heat and, when the mixture is cool enough to handle, ladle it into a food processor and blend to a smooth puree. Meanwhile, bring milk to a simmer in a saucepan. Combine mushroom puree and milk in a bowl, stirring to mix. For extra smoothness, or if leek fibers are present, pass soup through a fine sieve. Adjust seasoning to taste. If soup is not hot enough to serve, reheat gently in a saucepan without allowing it to boil.

4. To serve, transfer soup to warm serving bowls or individual tureens, then garnish as desired.

Chef's tip: If you used dried *cèpes,* the soaking liquid may be used to replace an equivalent quantity of stock.

SALMON BURGERS

Serves 3; 200 calories per serving
Preparation time: 20 minutes

Ingredients
6$^1/_2$ oz. fillet of salmon
3$^1/_2$ oz. peeled langoustines (or jumbo shrimp)
3$^1/_2$ oz. peeled prawns
$^1/_2$ an egg white (about $^1/_2$ oz.)
1$^1/_4$ oz. plain nonfat yogurt
1$^1/_2$ tsp. finely grated lime zest
1$^1/_2$ tsp. coarsely ground green peppercorns
1 oz. salmon roe
1 tsp. olive oil
Salt and pepper, to taste
3 lemon wedges, for garnish (optional)
3 sprigs of watercress or small salad leaves, for garnish (optional)

Instructions
1. Dice salmon, langoustines, and prawns into $^1/_4$-inch pieces.
2. In a large mixing bowl, whisk egg white until it forms a very soft peak, then whisk in yogurt, lime zest, and peppercorns. Add diced seafood, and mix with a fork. Add roe, and mix again gently to distribute the ingredients. Taste and adjust the seasoning, then briefly stir again.
3. Put three food rings, 3$^1/_2$ to 4 inches in diameter, on a baking sheet or tray covered with greaseproof or parchment paper. Spoon fish

mixture into the rings, and level the tops. Transfer baking sheet to the refrigerator for 1 hour to allow the burger mixture to firm slightly.

4. When ready to cook the burgers, remove them from the refrigerator. Heat olive oil in a nonstick frying pan. Carefully lift away food rings, then lift each burger with a spatula and gently slide it into the pan, easing it off the spatula with a knife if necessary. Cook burgers for 2 minutes on each side, turning carefully with the spatula.

———◆———

CHICKEN BREASTS STUFFED WITH LEMONY HERBS

Serves 4; 240 calories per serving
Preparation time: 50 minutes (worth every minute)

Ingredients
2 tbsp. *fromage blanc* or nonfat Greek yogurt
1 tsp. finely chopped chives
1 tsp. finely chopped flat-leaf parsley
1 tsp. lemon confit, cut into $1/4$-inch pieces
Salt and pepper
2 chicken breasts, skin removed
$1^1/4$ to $1^2/3$ cups White Vegetable Sauce (recipe follows)
$4^1/2$ oz. snow peas
2 artichoke hearts, fresh, preserved, or frozen, thawed
1 clove unpeeled garlic
1 tsp. olive oil
7 oz. fresh tagliatelle or fettucine
Sprigs of tarragon, for garnish

Instructions
1. For the stuffing, mix together *fromage blanc*, chives, parsley, and lemon confit. Season to taste with salt and pepper.
2. To fill chicken breasts, cut two pieces of plastic wrap, each large enough to comfortably wrap a breast. Using a small knife, ease open the natural running pocket of each breast lengthwise, leaving it closed at each end. Season chicken inside and out. Divide filling between the pockets, and close them. Wrap breasts tightly in plastic wrap, and set aside in the refrigerator.

3. Boil water beneath a steamer basket for the chicken and a saucepan of salted water for the pasta. Heat White Vegetable Sauce and keep it warm, preferably in a double boiler.

4. To prepare and cook the vegetables, cut snow peas diagonally at regular intervals to make diamond shapes. Drain artichoke hearts and dice them. Sweat diced artichokes along with the clove of garlic over gentle heat in a saucepan coated with olive oil for about 2 minutes. Add peas and cover. Sweat gently for about 10 minutes, shaking the saucepan or stirring occasionally to prevent sticking.

5. While vegetables are sweating, steam wrapped chicken breasts for about 6 minutes. Remove breasts with a spatula, and leave to cool briefly. Meanwhile, cook fresh pasta in simmering water until al dente, then drain.

6. Remove and discard garlic from the vegetables. Remove plastic wrap from chicken breasts, and cut each breast into four to six slices.

7. Prepare four warm plates. Make a nest of pasta on each plate, and arrange slices of stuffed chicken breasts alongside. Add vegetable garnish and a small pool of White Vegetable Sauce. (You may add some finely chopped mixed herbs to the sauce at the last moment, if you wish.) Decorate with a sprig of tarragon. Serve immediately.

WHITE VEGETABLE SAUCE

Serves 20; 19 calories per $1/4$-oz. serving
The base of this versatile sauce is a white vegetable liaison.

Ingredients

1 tsp. olive oil
7 oz. chopped leeks
7 oz. white button mushrooms, wiped and chopped
$5^{1}/_{2}$ oz. potatoes, peeled and chopped
$3^{1}/_{2}$ oz. chopped onions (I use yellow onions)
$3^{1}/_{2}$ oz. chopped celeriac
2 oz. cauliflower, trimmed and chopped
$1/_{4}$ oz. chopped garlic
$2^{1}/_{8}$ cups chicken stock
Salt and pepper
Pinch of nutmeg (optional)
$3/_{4}$ cup 2 percent milk
$1/_{4}$ cup stock (vegetable or chicken)

Instructions

1. Heat olive oil in a large saucepan on medium heat. Add vegetables, cover, and sweat gently for 2 minutes without coloring. Add garlic and chicken stock. Season, cover, and allow to simmer gently for 20 minutes or until flavors have combined.
2. Transfer sauce to a food processor and blend to a smooth, fine puree. Taste and adjust seasonings if needed; add nutmeg, if using.
3. Blend $3\frac{1}{2}$ oz. of sauce with milk and stock. Pass blended mixture through a fine sieve.
4. Heat and adjust seasonings before serving.

GARDEN-FRESH LEMON SORBET

Serves 4; 70 to 310 calories per serving, depending on sweetener
Preparation time: 40 minutes

Ingredients

4 organic lemons
$2\frac{1}{8}$ cups, plus 3 tbsp. water
6 heaping tbsp., plus 1 pinch sweetener*
7 oz. fresh raspberries, plus extra for decoration
4 small mixed bunches of fresh verbena, mint, and rosemary

Instructions

1. To make the syrup for the sorbet, zest three of the lemons over a sauce-pan. Add $2\frac{1}{8}$ cups water and 6 heaping tablespoons of sweetener, then bring mixture to a boil. Once boiling, remove saucepan from heat.
2. Cut all four lemons in half, and juice them. Stir juice into the warm syrup.
3. Transfer syrup to an ice-cream maker and churn to a soft consistency. Alternatively, put mixture in a shallow freezing tray and stir thoroughly every half hour with a fork. The sorbet will be ready after several hours when it has a soft, scoopable consistency. Put sorbet in an airtight container, and freeze until ready to serve.
4. Put raspberries and 3 tablespoons of water in the bowl of a food processor, and puree. Taste, and add a pinch of sweetener if required. For a smooth coulis, pass the puree through a fine sieve and discard pips. Pour the coulis into an airtight container, and place in the refrigerator until needed.
5. Prepare four chilled shallow dessert bowls or glass dishes. Remove sorbet from the freezer, and scoop out each portion using two

dessert spoons, passing the sorbet between the spoons to make oval quenelle shapes. Put one in each bowl. Drizzle a small amount of raspberry coulis over each helping. Add a few fresh raspberries, and decorate with a small bunch of fresh verbena, mint, and rosemary. Serve immediately.

The choice of sweeteners for the sorbet, with final calorie counts per serving:
Aspartame: 70; **Fructose:** 175; **Xylitol:** 210; **Honey:** 250; **Sugar:** 310 (Michel Guérard uses fructose; I use xylitol.)

Note: Michel Guérard serves *cuisine minceur* desserts with teaspoons, never dessert spoons because, as he says, the small spoons force us to slow down and savor the sweet experience. Then, at least in my case, a special tisane (herbal tea) was the final flourish to the exquisite meals.

FRAMBOISE CONFITURE (RASPBERRY JAM)

This was a special recipe given to me by Michel Guérard's daughter, Eléonore, so I do not have the calorie count. Let's simply agree that it fits perfectly into the *cuisine minceur régime*. I can tell you that it is delicious and that its simple preparation was my first foray into making *confiture*.

Ingredients
2.2 lbs. (1 kilo) fresh or frozen raspberries
2/3 cup xylitol
1 1/2 Tbsp. apple pectin
2 organic lemons, juiced

Instructions
1. In a saucepan, heat raspberries until boiling. (Stir and watch carefully—I'm speaking from experience.)
2. Mix the xylitol with the apple pectin.
3. Pour the xylitol-and-pectin mixture into the raspberries, and cook on low heat for about 20 minutes.
4. Remove from stove, and add lemon juice.
5. Let cool. As the mixture cools, it will jellify.
6. Store in the refrigerator.
NOTE: Eléonore didn't tell me how long it can be kept in the refrigerator. All I know is it disappears very quickly *chez nous*. It's wonderful on vanilla ice cream.

First published in the United States of America in 2018
by Rizzoli Ex Libris, an imprint of
Rizzoli International Publications, Inc.
300 Park Avenue South
New York, NY 10010
www.rizzoliusa.com

Illustrations on front cover and pages 3, 25, 33, 55, 79, 98, 105, 109, 113,
121, 142, 153, 159, 160, 175, 179, 189, 198, 202, 205, 211, 214, 239 by Sujean Rim.
Graphics from Jardin de Sophie by KLUGE + GRAN. Used with permission.
Grateful acknowledgment is made to Michel Guérard for permission to
reprint the recipes on pages 250–255.

2018 2019 2020 2021 / 10 9 8 7 6 5 4 3 2 1

Distributed in the U.S. trade by Random House, New York

Printed in the United States of America

ISBN-13: 978-0-8478-6305-1

Library of Congress Catalog Control Number: 2018948850

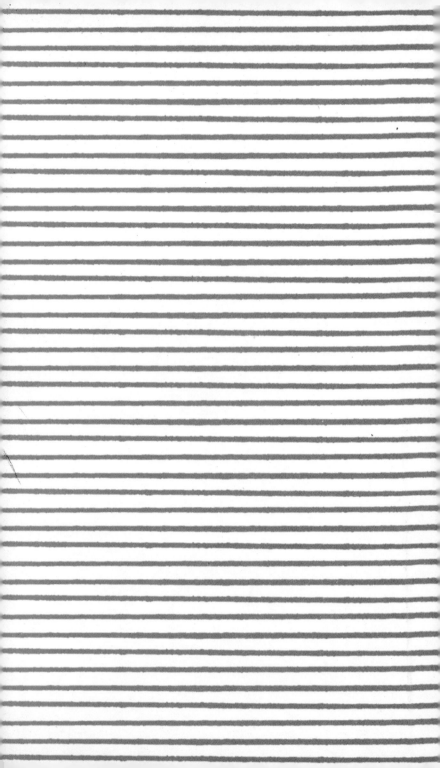